THE GIFT OF A

Peaceful Death

Kathryn F. Weymouth, PhD

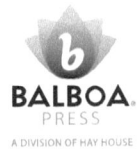

BALBOA.
PRESS

A DIVISION OF HAY HOUSE

Balboa Press books may be ordered through booksellers or by contacting:

Balboa Press
A Division of Hay House
1663 Liberty Drive
Bloomington, IN 47403
www.balboapress.com
1 (877) 407-4847

Because of the dynamic nature of the Internet, any web addresses or links contained in this book may have changed since publication and may no longer be valid. The views expressed in this work are solely those of the author and do not necessarily reflect the views of the publisher, and the publisher hereby disclaims any responsibility for them.

The author of this book does not dispense medical advice or prescribe the use of any technique as a form of treatment for physical, emotional, or medical problems without the advice of a physician, either directly or indirectly. The intent of the author is only to offer information of a general nature to help you in your quest for emotional and spiritual well-being. In the event you use any of the information in this book for yourself, which is your constitutional right, the author and the publisher assume no responsibility for your actions.

Any people depicted in stock imagery provided by Thinkstock are models, and such images are being used for illustrative purposes only.
Certain stock imagery © Thinkstock.

Print information available on the last page.

ISBN: 978-1-5043-8193-2 (sc)
ISBN: 978-1-5043-8194-9 (hc)
ISBN: 978-1-5043-8212-0 (e)

Library of Congress Control Number: 2017908935

Balboa Press rev. date: 06/29/2017

This book is dedicated to every person who so graciously agreed
to be interviewed and answered my many questions . . .

To every person who came before them who were
instrumental in supporting and training them to
become the very special professionals that they are,
dedicated to humanity and the relief of suffering . . .

And to all the people who will benefit from knowing about,
receiving, or giving the healing techniques described in this book.

Acknowledgments

It may seem strange to acknowledge forces unseen for this book and previous ones, but I must. With my first book, *What Obituaries Don't Tell You: Conversations About Life and Death,* it was as if an idea fell out of the sky into my mind, took hold, and wouldn't let go until I agreed to bring it to fruition.

My second book, *A Way Through: Healing from Loss,* is a workbook that was a logical follow-up to the first book although it might not have been written were it not for the not-so-subtle urgings from my earthly friends who said, "You need to do this."

The book that you have in your hands now was, again, an idea that would not let go, and every person except one whom I contacted for interviews said "yes" and were eager to share their knowledge and experiences with readers. The ease of finding the right people and their enthusiasm was a message to me that forces beyond my capabilities were aligned in favor of this project. I had tried to do research for a different book before embarking on this one and got absolutely nowhere. People I contacted didn't respond, those who did were retired or not interested, so I finally had to admit that this was not the project I was meant to be undertaking and I set it aside.

I had originally thought that this book, *The Gift of a Peaceful Death,* would be my fourth book, but obviously I was wrong. I believe that each of us receives messages from whatever those unseen forces are, sometimes as a gentle push, an inspired thought, serendipitous events, someone's belief in us, a passion that is burning to be expressed, or, as in the case with my project that was a no-go, nothing works.

Whenever a major new idea or life direction occurred, my experience was one of feeling as if a string was attached to the middle of my chest and was pulling me toward whatever that new thing was. This force wasn't me, it wasn't anyone else telling me I should do such and such, this was an invisible force that I could follow or resist, it was up to me. I don't remember resisting for very long, though, in any of the situations in which I experienced this as a strong force that would not go away.

Did I experience this force with the book that did not come into fruition? I know that I was very curious about the topic, I was interested in meeting and interviewing people and learning more about them and their cultures, but the energy of it seemed more in my head than in my heart, and it seems that it's from the heart first, and the head second, that is the dynamic of the force that I have described.

So in listening to my internal guidance, which I talk about in the Introduction, and following that energetic pull, here I am speaking to you about relieving suffering by using techniques that are still not well known in our Western world. I am adding my voice, and the voices of everyone I interviewed, to others who want people to know about complementary and alternative modalities that can be used in conjunction with their standard medical care for an integrative approach to health and wellness, or in terminal illness and end-of-life care which is the focus of this book.

Some people say that there is something noble and spiritual about suffering, but I am not one of them. I think the purpose of suffering is to learn how not to suffer, and if the lesson is needed, to learn compassion for those who suffer. If you think about the people over the centuries who have dedicated their lives to learning how to reduce or eliminate suffering, you are looking at a very large number of people, both well-known or laboring in relative obscurity, and the work goes on.

It is hard work to experience your own suffering, and to watch other people suffer, and when in that state we are constantly looking for ways that will provide relief. This is exactly the focus of this book. If something has inspired you to read this book, I believe that unknown force for good is at work. Be open to where it may lead you. It could change your life, and the lives of others.

Kathryn F. Weymouth, PhD
Portland, Oregon
May, 2017

Table of Contents

Introduction

This, my third book on dying and death, was inspired by Anne's story, the first story in *What Obituaries Don't Tell You: Conversations About Life and Death* (Weymouth, 2013).

Anne was called by her friend and former nursing school roommate after she was diagnosed with ovarian cancer, wanting to know if she was receiving the best care from the best doctors. Anne checked with a relative who was a doctor, determined that she was in good hands, and offered to do energy healing with her to help cope with the fear and anxiety and ease the physical symptoms from the cancer and the treatments. Reluctant at first to take Anne up on her offer of Healing Touch, Betsy said yes before long and the story that ensued is a beautiful example of what energy healing can do for the recipient, the provider, family members, co-workers, and friends.

I learned so much from the people who graciously told me their stories for *What Obituaries Don't Tell You*. Almost every day something would happen that would remind me of one or more of the stories, the people who told me the stories, and the lives and deaths of the people whom the stories were about. Friends kept asking me what my next book was going to be about and I thought they must be crazy; they had no idea how much work writing a book is. But in short order I knew exactly what my next book would be about. Anne and Betsy's story kept coming to my mind and I thought, "The seeds of a book are there, showing how using complementary and alternative methods can be used to ease pain and anxiety and help create a peaceful death." At first I thought the book would focus only on Healing Touch, the practitioners, the uses, and the outcomes, but as you will see the research broadened to include much more than that.

Kathryn F. Weymouth, PhD

A motivating factor for this book, *A Peaceful Death*, is that I am a Healing Touch Certified Practitioner and have experienced first hand the power of this gentle work to make remarkable differences in people's lives. I was certified on July 6, 1997, #571 with the required recertification every five years since to maintain certified status. I am one of the few with a PhD in psychology rather than credentialed in the nursing field. Healing Touch entered my life via a guest speaker at a small group session of people whom I would term spiritual explorers when our facilitator invited a friend of hers from graduate school to do a presentation for us. Sharon Scandrett-Hibdon, RN, PhD, FNP spoke to us about an energy healing method that she was instrumental in developing and which recently had begun certifying students who successfully completed the extensive training, mentored internship, and certification review.

This was not the first time I had been introduced to energy healing. Fourteen years earlier I had received training in a healing method developed by a man who combined several techniques he had learned and some that he developed, but there was no credentialing involved, and his course was offered to only a few people in his hometown. It was through my association with Dan, however, that I fell in love with energy healing and witnessed how effective it can be. Effective seems such a lame word to use to describe what I saw then, and what I have experienced since, but it will suffice for now and I will let the reader judge for him or herself and substitute any word that may more accurately capture the essence of the experience. Here is what happened.

In the fall of 1977 my mother was stopped at a stoplight when a drunk, going between 80 and 100 miles an hour slammed into the rear of her car. Several witnesses told the police that they had been forced off the road by this driver, but my mother did not see him coming and could probably have done nothing to avoid him even if she had. Her car burst into flames and through an heroic effort she was able to lie down on the seat, pull her knees up to her chest and kick the door open. She jumped out through a wall of flames and rolled out onto the street to extinguish her burning clothes. She was taken to the burn unit at a local hospital where she spent the next several weeks.

Even though she was getting good care there, I knew that more could be done to ease her pain. I'm not even sure how I knew, I just knew that something underneath that broad umbrella labeled "healing" could help her. I inquired around town, asking if anyone knew a healer, and was given Dan's name. He said that he would be happy to visit my mom and give her a treatment, and said that he would bring some of his students with him and invited both my sister, Jennifer, and me to participate.

If you have ever visited anyone in a burn unit you know that you have to be very careful about keeping the environment as free of contaminants as possible, so this required that we gown up and put on face masks and gloves before entering her room. Dan, his four students, and my sister and I gathered around my mother's bed, we went into a peaceful, calm, meditative state, held our hands out toward Mom, and with gentle energy from our hands and healing intention in our hearts and minds, we projected healing energy toward her. After about fifteen minutes Dan said that was enough and we all left. Mom didn't say goodbye because she was sound asleep.

The next day I went to visit her and the first thing she asked was "What did you do last night?" I thought, "Oh, oh, am I in trouble," so I simply said, "Why do you ask?" She said, "I remember you coming in and before long I was floating above my body looking at everybody. The room was filled with purple light, and at one point one of the women had to leave because she said she was too hot. Then I fell asleep and slept for eight hours with no pain." At that point I knew I had witnessed and participated in a miracle. Sleeping all night with no pain just a few days after being burned over twenty percent of your body and requiring skin grafts? Even the pain medication couldn't provide that much relief. And she was right; one of the women did have to leave the room because she was too hot.

After this experience I simply had to know more and I was on the road to becoming an energy healer but I didn't know it, and it didn't happen right away. As a mother of two young sons, and still a few years away from opening my private practice, I had a few opportunities to practice what I had learned from Dan, but not many.

Seven years later I was introduced to Therapeutic Touch and took classes from my good friend, Anthony. He was an excellent instructor and a person who fascinated me because he seemed perfectly capable of using both sides of his brain equally well. Career-wise he was an engineer and helped develop a portable pump for diabetics, but in his personal life he was what I would describe as tuned in to the subtle realms of energy, intuition, and healing. It was in his class that I learned the importance of intention, and that with too much ego involved the energy that is transmitted can have a negative rather than a positive effect. During one of our exercises I got very sick from the energy being transmitted to me by my practice partner and had to have Anthony put me back together, so to speak, before I could leave the class and drive home safely. That was a lesson that I never forgot because it showed me the power of intentionally directed energy, and it also showed me how important it is to get out of the way and let the pure healing energy simply flow through you. But as much as I loved the healing work, and by then I had opened my private counseling practice, healing didn't fit in very well because I had not yet identified myself as a healer, either to myself or my clients, so that was not an expected part of the work that I offered.

Over the years I have had to conclude that I am not completely in control of my life because it seemed that whatever the forces are that influence a person were not done with me yet, and once again, seven years later, I was introduced to Healing Touch. During that presentation by Sandra Scandrett-Hibdon a little voice in my head kept saying, "You are going to do this, and you are going all the way through the program and get certified." The other part of my mind was saying "But it is so much work! Three or four years before certification, and everything that I have to do to reach that goal! Besides, I have back problems and how am I going to be able to stand at a massage table for hours at a time to give healing sessions?" These objections had no impact at all on the voice that just kept calmly informing me that I was going to do this, so I did.

Saying "Yes" changed my life. My back was healed and I learned skills that I have used over the years to facilitate healing for others for many different kinds of problems. There are times at the close of a session that I feel so strongly the sacredness of the work that I give thanks that this work found me and kept knocking at my door until I said yes and fully committed.

Because I know the beauty and potential of energy healing, Anne's story kept coming into my mind and would not let go. Her work with Betsy is such a powerful example of how much good can be done with the healing work that I knew I wanted to share this with the world. Yes, Betsy died from the cancer, and nothing can prevent the grief of such a loss, but as Anne said it was as good a death as could be expected under the circumstances. Betsy was able to stay at home under hospice care; her husband, her children, and her mother were actively involved in the care; the hospital chaplain did a beautiful blessing that involved Anne and the entire family; and Healing Touch provided relief and compassionate presence in which conversations of deep significance could take place. Betsy's husband said, "The Healing Touch that Betsy received from Anne was the first kind of spirituality I saw awaken in her, and the first time I ever saw Betsy put any credence into that kind of activity. She found real benefit and comfort in it. I could see the change in her, she was so much more relaxed, more at ease, at peace. You could really feel that. Anne created a very calming environment, and it was comforting to me to see Betsy comforted."

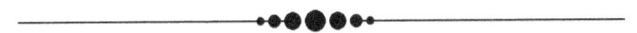

A peaceful death is the most precious gift that we can offer a loved one.

When I read this sentence in Alberto Villoldo's book, *Shaman, Healer, Sage* (Villoldo, 2000) it struck a deep chord in me. When I read it the first time I had no idea that in a few years I would be researching, writing, and counseling about dying and death, but I never forgot it and it continues to reverberate through my work – the gift of a peaceful death. So even though at first I thought it was a crazy idea to write another book the pieces started coming together: write about resources that few people even know exist, resources for pain and anxiety reduction, and helping ease into a peaceful death.

At the beginning of my research I thought I would just be interviewing Healing Touch practitioners who had completed the certification process, but it soon became apparent that the scope of the research needed to be broadened considerably. Most certified practitioners are nurses as the program was originally offered through the American Holistic Nurses Association (AHNA), so I started my interviews with nurses and with the very first interview I learned that my focus was much too narrow, that I needed to add the use of music, aromatherapy, massage, acupuncture, and silent or shared prayer to the list of modalities as many of them used these in conjunction with Healing Touch. A hospital chaplain didn't think he was a good candidate to be interviewed because he wasn't certified, but what he had learned in the first level of Healing Touch training was enough that he was able to benefit his patients tremendously. Almost everybody that I interviewed said, "You need to interview so and so," and they would give me the name of someone else doing comfort care for the dying. Every practitioner I contacted was eager to share their experiences because of the benefit that their particular expertise provided to patients. The modalities represented in this book are Healing Touch, massage therapy, acupuncture, essential oils/aromatherapy, music therapy, and palliative care. Interviews were done with nurses, a nursing professor, a hospital chaplain, a hospice chaplain, massage therapists, an acupuncturist, the president of a college of healthcare and expert in essential oils and aromatherapy, a music therapist, and palliative care physicians.

The stories in the book illustrate the blending of Western mainstream medicine with complementary modalities. The terminology is beginning to change from Complementary and Alternative Medicine (CAM) to Complementary and Integrative Medicine, although the acronym CAM is still in standard usage. I am pleased to see the integrative medicine terminology and practice gaining wider visibility. I have long said that when Western medicine and complementary medicine can join forces we will have a model that combines the masculine and feminine, the yin and the yang, and therefore treats the whole person.

Western medicine is more masculine with its use of machines, surgeries, pharmaceuticals that often have serious side effects, and the brief, often impersonal encounters between physician, patient, and family members.

Complementary modalities express more feminine qualities as they are typically softer, slower, non-invasive, non-pharmaceutical, and more relational. What one can do the other cannot do, and each approach has its own place in medicine, each practitioner has chosen his or her profession because of the way they personally want to alleviate suffering, and each can be a complement to the other.

Often patients and families do not benefit from complementary modalities because they do not know about them, they have heard about them but are skeptical as to any benefits they may offer, and in some medical settings physicians are not allowed to mention them or don't believe in them but may have no objections if the patient or family asks for them.

One of the arguments made against complementary and alternative care is that it prevents the patient from getting the treatment that would be most beneficial to them. In illnesses and accidents in which recovery is unlikely and it is simply a matter of time before death occurs, it would be rare for a person to completely eschew mainstream interventions although it does happen because of personal beliefs or the failure of what has been tried and has not worked. There will always be the question of what to do, what is best, which might be summed up by asking when more is less and less is more.

The purpose of this book, then, is to let people know that these healing modalities exist, that they are professionally recognized with educational and credentialing requirements, when and how they are used, what they do, and their role in complementary and integrative medicine. Once you know you can ask for them for yourself and your loved ones, and maybe be inspired to become a practitioner yourself.

Healing Touch Overview

In the Introduction I referred to Anne's story in my book *What Obituaries Don't Tell You: Conversations About Life and Death,* which was the impetus for this book. I want to share excerpts of the story with you but before I do that it will be helpful to know more about Healing Touch itself.

Application

Simply put, Healing Touch is a method of hands-on-healing – although it is often done without touching the body – that enhances the body's ability to heal, calms and clears the mind, promotes positive emotional states, and aids in receptivity to spiritual connection. If you are a parent who has ever soothed your child with touch, or comforted them with your presence and words, you have practiced healing touch. The difference between healing touch and Healing Touch is that the latter is a system of interventions that are given for specific purposes, and to become a Healing Touch practitioner requires five levels of course work, hands-on training and practice, followed by a certification process. In my research (Weymouth, 2002)[1] the top ten purposes for which practitioners used Healing Touch were: pain reduction, anxiety and stress reduction, relaxation, to maintain wellness, to accelerate healing from a disease or illness, to accelerate post-operative healing, to deal with emotional trauma, to ease the dying process, to ease depression, for insomnia, and for respiratory problems. But as you will see in Anne's story, it also facilitates meaningful conversations, allows family members and friends to be involved in the treatments in loving and gentle ways, and provides a safe space to celebrate life and face death.

History

Healing Touch was founded by Janet Mentgen, BSN, RN, (1938-2005) based upon and incorporating her education and training in nursing, her nursing practice, several energy healing modalities in which she was trained, techniques that she developed herself, and teaching.

For nine years, from 1980 to 1989, she used the techniques in her private healing practice, and at the urging of some colleagues began to develop the curriculum which became the Healing Touch Program™. In 1989, the president of the American Holistic Nurses Association (AHNA), Lynn Keegan, asked Mentgen if she would like to offer the Healing Touch course as a certificate program. The nurses credited with developing the Healing Touch Program™ are Janet Mentgen, Dorothea Hover-Kramer, EdD, RN, Sharon Scandrett-Hibdon, RN, PhD and Myra Tovey, RN, BS.

Course certification was granted in 1990 when Scandrett-Hibdon was president of AHNA and the rest of the group were on the Board of Directors. Certification of practitioners and instructors began in 1993. In 1996 the AHNA took up the issue of whether or not they would certify practitioners who were not nurses. Mentgen was committed to training anyone who was interested in the work and would practice under the ethical standards of the program, whereas the AHNA felt that certifying anyone not a nurse overstepped their mandate as a nursing organization. The decision was made that AHNA would continue to endorse the program but certification would come through a new organization. In 1996 Healing Touch International (HTI) was incorporated as the program's certifying body with headquarters in Lakewood, Colorado.

Eventually the program became two entities: Healing Touch Program™, www.healingtouchprogram.com and Healing Beyond Borders, Education and Certifying the Healing Touch.®, www.healingbeyondborders.org Both programs use Mentgen's teachings and levels toward certification, but only the Healing Touch Program™ is accredited by the National Commission for Certifying Agencies (NCCA), making it the only exclusively energy medicine education program to have achieved national accreditation. The

Healing Touch Program™ is endorsed by the American Holistic Nurses Association (AHNA), The Canadian Holistic Nurses Association (CHNA), accredited as a provider of continuing nursing education by the American Nurses Credentialing Center's Commission of Accreditation (ANCC), and approved by the National Certification Board for Therapeutic Massage and Bodywork (NCBTMB) as a continuing education approved provider. Healing Beyond Borders® is endorsed by the American Holistic Nurses Association (AHNA), approved by the National Certification Board for Therapeutic Massage and Bodywork (NCBTMB), and approved as a California Nurses provider.

Requirements for certification

To become a certified practitioner five levels of education, training, and hands-on-experience is required. The mentored apprenticeship, of approximately one to two years post-class room time and application and practice of techniques, is followed by submission of qualifying materials to a panel of examiners. Once certification has been achieved, recertification is required every five years to maintain certified status. For recertification in the Healing Touch Program™, proof of 75 hours of continuing education is required: recertification requirements in Healing Beyond Borders® is essentially the same. As an adjunct to other health care modalities, Healing Touch is offered in many hospitals, hospices, health care facilities, and private counseling and healing practices. Many communities offer regularly scheduled free sessions at hospitals, churches, homeless shelters, and other gathering places.

The specific interventions that are mentioned in the interviews are not described in detail because this is copyrighted information and would not be of great value to the reader without being trained in them. However, there are YouTube videos that discuss Healing Touch and demonstrate techniques, and thanks to Janet Mentgen and her vision of having somebody in every household know how to do energy healing you can sign up for courses with the Healing Touch Program™ or Healing Beyond Borders®.

Summary

Anyone who is trained in Healing Touch has at heart a deeply held desire to ease suffering and provide a type of healing that is rarely present in modern-day medicine. I often think of American Medical Association (AMA) medicine as masculine with its machines, pills, and surgeries, and complementary and alternative practices as feminine, with its compassionate presence, touch, and other modalities you will read about in this book. If we can combine these approaches more often than is being done now we would have holistic and integrative medicine that would benefit patients, clients, families, and professionals.

Although the primary focus of this book is on terminal illnesses and end-of-life care, the techniques can be used at any point in a person's life for enhanced wellness and relief of suffering. When I asked the professionals whom I interviewed how they thought complementary and alternative modalities can be integrated into mainstream medicine, they said it will happen when patients in large enough numbers ask for it, i.e., patient demand. Once you read about the techniques and their benefits described in this book I hope it inspires you to ask for them on behalf of your loved ones, your patients and clients, and for yourself.

---

1. Comparing the Efficacy of Healing Touch and Chiropractic Adjustment in Treating Chronic Low Back Pain: A Pilot Study. Master's Thesis (2002), Saybrook Graduate School. Research summary available at kweymouth.com

Anne's Story
Nurse
Nursing Instructor
Healing Touch Certified Practitioner

Introduction

The following are excerpts from Anne's story from my book *What Obituaries Don't Tell You: Conversations About Life and Death.* It is this story and my personal experience with Healing Touch, both as a recipient and a practitioner, that made me want to share this work and other complementary and alternative methods with people who are suffering, people who want to help relieve suffering, and everyone who wants to have a peaceful death.

Interview

I got home after midnight, and there was a message on my machine asking for my help. I rushed over to the hospital where my roommate from nursing school and long-term friend had just been diagnosed with stage 4 colon cancer and needed to make some fast decisions, hopefully the right ones, about what to do next. One of my relatives is a doctor and she wanted me to consult with him. As it turned out, she was being seen by the best physicians, which was her greatest concern at the time: "Am I being treated by the right doctors? Can I trust their recommendations?"

The cancer was a surprise. She had been having symptoms for six months, but they were all upper GI symptoms; dyspepsia, heartburn, that kind of thing. All of the work-ups and diagnostics were for upper GI problems, and they were looking particularly at the probability of gallbladder problems.

Even though Betsy and I were both nurses, our interests and approaches to medicine took some divergent paths. By this time I had become interested in complementary and alternative medicine, whereas Betsy was very pragmatic, no-nonsense, scientific approach only kind of gal. I had been learning Healing Touch and offered it to her for pain and anxiety management, but her response was "thanks but no thanks." So I just said, "Let me know. You may get to the point where you might want to try this."

Soon after her first surgery I was visiting her at the hospital, and she was in pain crisis and emotional crisis because of all the decisions that had to be made around chemo and treatment, it was just a highly emotional situation. So finally she agreed to the Healing Touch, and I did the treatment right there in the hospital. She liked it, and that's what started the deeper connection between us and regular Healing Touch treatments right up until she died ten months later. I did energy work on her every day for the last ten days of her life, and actually kind of moved in with them for the last three days.

When it became obvious that she wasn't going to recover, Betsy decided that she wanted to die at home. Her husband and the hospice nurse set up the environment, the equipment, and the medications exactly as he wanted. He and their daughter learned how to run the machines and deliver the IV medications. I served more in a support and advisory role, like talking to the family about pain management, suggesting when it seemed advisable to consult with hospice on that and other issues, being the go-between for family members, friends and colleagues, telling the family when the signs were suggesting that the end was near, these sorts of things.

That whole question about good death, bad death . . . it was probably as good as many of them get. Really, the only thing I can say that was bad about it was that it was a 44-year-old woman who really was not ready to leave life and her family and her roles. For both of us the question: "Why does this have to happen?" It was so sad, so sad. The hardest thing for me about Betsy's death was she was never ready. You know how you read and you talk about the good death, one where the person comes to terms with it, they're ready to leave, they've taken care of all their unfinished business, and it's this peaceful death. Well, that's not what I felt for her. Her family might say differently, but some of her last words were, "This is not fair, I am not ready to leave you guys." And you know, I came to terms with that pretty easily because of course I was thinking of myself. We're the same age, two kids, like looking in the mirror. I would also be thinking it's not fair. There's a lot in life that's not fair, but I would still be thinking that, and thinking "I don't want to be leaving here."

From a professional perspective, Betsy's death was the kind of experience I would strive for, for patients, the kinds of outcomes I would look for. I don't think she was in a lot of pain. She had incredible love and support, and except for her ambivalence about being ready to go, I think it went really well. So, in terms of creating a comfortable, and I would say spiritual environment for somebody who was leaving, it was pretty darn good. Both Betsy and her husband were people who needed to have control over their environment. They needed information, and then they needed permission to make the decisions about what was best for them. From a health care perspective it's important to remember when you're interfacing with people who are coping with whatever, is to not draw conclusions without enough data, and to really sit back and let people be individuals unless it's harmful. When Betsy was in pain or agitated, the family and I would discuss what we should do, and I would always say, "What do you think she would want? What do you want for her? She trusted us to manage her symptoms at home." We knew what she wanted, she wanted to be kept comfortable.

What some would consider to be a good death would be totally different from Betsy's experience. For example, I've always believed that people should not die alone, but there are probably some people who would choose that. In fact, it's not uncommon that a person will hang on until everybody has gone for lunch, or coffee, or a break of some kind, and then the person dies while everybody is out of the room.

Even though Betsy fought until the very end, she was a full participant in plans for the final stages of dying, and plans for the memorial service. During the last couple of weeks of her life, when she was still aware and coherent, her husband got a big piece of wood and a frame, and brought out the shoebox of family photos. They went through it and made a collage of just their family, just the four of them. On the back he took excerpts from cards that people had written to her at the end, mostly people from her work, who talked about who she was. That was very healing, and it turned out to be a phenomenal picture. Her hospital bed was right in the dining room, and the area where people worked on the collage was right there where you went from the living room into the dining room. It was in that area, too, that Betsy's daughter, son, and his girlfriend and I sat on the floor and made safety pin bracelets. So we had the collage out, we had the beads out, it gave us something to do. We all wore our beaded bracelets at the memorial service.

When they came and took the body away, that was really hard. I wish it had been done differently. At our local hospice, when someone dies, the staff and the family walk the body out to the car, they stay with the body. We just stayed in the living room, looking out the window, just holding onto each other as they put the body into the back of the van. It was a very cold experience, really hard, and then she was gone. Looking back, I wish we had walked the body out, having it be a little more ceremonial, a more reverent transition.

Betsy was not religious, but her mother is Catholic and wanted her to have last rites, which was not anything Betsy wanted. So Mary, the hospital chaplain who knew her quite well through her professional role, mediated a meeting with Betsy and her mom to come to some sort of compromise, and did just an incredible job. What Betsy agreed to was that when she was getting close to the end we would call Mary and she would come to the house and do a ritual with us. The ritual was just this profound experience for everyone, because everyone at that point was ready for her to let go. I don't know about Betsy, I have my hunch that she wasn't ready, but everyone else was telling her "Mom, Betsy, we'll be okay, you need to go, we're going to be okay."

Mary did this blessing where we talked about who Betsy was, as a mother, a friend, a nurse, all her different roles. Then she went through parts of her body and invited all of us who were there, her husband, her two children, her mother, and me, to bless that body part if we felt drawn to do so. So you know, it was her eyes, her ears, her hands, her feet. It was very, very intimate, a wonderful way for the kids to say goodbye to their mother. It really allowed them to touch her and be with her and really say what they wanted to say in a safe way, with people they trusted. It had been about 24 hours since Betsy had said anything, and during the blessing the subject of yellow roses came up. Her favorite were yellow roses, which she wanted at her memorial service, so yellow roses were mentioned at one point during the blessing. Betsy whispered, "Yellow roses are my favorite." I believe the ritual woke her up, she was there, she was connected in that moment to what was happening. And certainly I felt she was very connected in energetically through the whole experience. That was profound, and not the kind of thing I've ever seen happen in a hospital environment. Maybe it has and I just haven't seen it.

I had talked to Betsy's husband and children about the signs that would indicate the end was near, the mottling in the legs that indicate the circulation is shutting down, the lack of urine output, the changes in the breathing, and it was when we saw these signs that we called Mary to come and do the blessing. So we called about 11:00 at night, she came and did the blessing, and by the time we were done everyone was exhausted. I said, "If you guys are comfortable, I'll stay awake at her bedside and I'll wake you when I think she is ready to go." Her son had lit candles throughout the whole house and we joked that we had better blow some of them out or else we would have a fire, but it was fun to see how the children created an environment for themselves and the family that was meaningful to them.

I sat in a chair next to Betsy's bed, trying to hold her hand, trying to stay awake and alert to when she needed medication and when she would be taking her last breaths. I had this sense that it would be like Betsy to want to go when we weren't all watching, so I had this ambivalence about letting that happen and also feeling like I needed to honor my trust with the family, that they wanted to be there. I kept my hand on her chest just lightly so I could sense changes. She didn't take a breath for like 15 seconds. I waited, she took another breath, and than I went and got everyone. They all came around and within a couple of minutes she took a couple more breaths, would stop breathing, then a breath, until finally there were no more breaths and she died at 6:00 in the morning. Her husband and children and I had already talked about how we would be able to tell energetically when her spirit left her body. We definitely didn't want to call for her to be picked up until her spirit had gone, and we had agreed to keep her as long as we felt comfortable. Hospice nurses tell you that you will know when you're ready to call for the body to be taken.

Were there gifts for me in this experience, working with Betsy as she was dying? Yes, many. Her death reminds me of how lucky I am, and not to take for granted a lot of things with my immediate family; our health, our relationships, our care for one another. When you say goodbye to each other you never know if that's going to be the last goodbye. Being a part of the blessing I just described, being able to help Betsy and her family as a friend and a professional, and even having my family be a part of her process was a gift. My kids learned an incredible amount. Our families would often have dinner together, and we would talk about her chemotherapy treatment, her hair and weight loss, and how much her appearance had changed. I don't want to say it became normal for them, but they achieved a level of comfort with it, and I value that.

But the biggest gift of all is that working with Betsy liberated my ambivalence about Healing Touch. It was through my work with her that I became a committed Healing Touch practitioner. Many times prior to working with Betsy I would ask myself, "Why am I doing this, why am I doing this?" And then I would get sucked right back in and guided toward doing the work. It was through working with Betsy's 10-month illness that it was hands-down, no question in my mind, the benefits of using this modality. It wasn't just the pain relief, helping with the anxiety, but it opened a more intimate communication channel between us. It was often after an energy treatment that she would have a conversation with me concerning something she needed to talk to her husband about. That was one of those powerful things of Healing Touch. Betsy was a good communicator, but not a -- how can I describe it –would not always initiate, didn't always speak her truth real well, didn't always express what was on her mind. She got to the point where she was talking pretty openly about the fact that she was going to be gone. She talked to me a lot in private about what she had hoped for the kids, what her fears were about how their dad would handle parenting the kids without her.

Healing Touch allowed a connection between Betsy's mom and her that would have been difficult otherwise. Her mother is very demonstrative in her love and affection, and wanted to touch and be near Betsy. In the last stages of cancer touching the person's body may cause pain, but Healing Touch can be done without touching, or by placing the hands only where it does not cause pain. I had her mother help with a session so she could participate and show her love and caring in ways that Betsy's body could accept.

A couple of months before Betsy died, two of her friends, past roommates, came to visit. They asked me if they could watch a Healing Touch treatment and Betsy said "sure." I'm doing the treatment, and I could tell they wanted to be involved. So I gave them some basic principles, and once they relaxed into the treatment and were part of the whole thing that was happening, they both started talking to her about what she meant to them. It was very healing for all three of them, all of us, really, to experience that. That was another gift Healing Touch provided, facilitating a closure experience for people. It was incredible.

Healing Touch Interviews

Mary[*]
Registered Nurse
Bachelor of Science
Holistic Nurse - Board Certified
Certified Healing Touch Practitioner and Instructor

Introduction

Mary is one of the original founders of Healing Touch. I was privileged to attend a workshop she gave in the beautiful Sun Valley area in Idaho, and she graciously granted me an interview while there. It was so interesting to hear about how the women who worked with Janet Mentgen to found The Healing Touch Program™ came together, how they dedicated so much time to the internal process of meditating about the vision and mission of the program, and the implementation of the work and the training of practitioners and instructors. It's not often that one gets to interview a person instrumental in developing and disseminating a program that has gone worldwide, touching the lives of thousands of people in profound ways.

Interview

My history with Healing Touch began in 1988 when I was appointed to the Holistic Nurses board after the north central regional director resigned. The Holistic Nurses conference was held in Colorado that year, and Janet Mentgen was voted holistic nurse of the year.

At our first board meeting I learned that Janet had a program on energy medicine that she was teaching at a community college in Colorado, and two other nurses had also studied energy work. You know how things happen, the four of us came together, started listening to what Janet was teaching, and when she found out that I had been studying with Brugh Joy[1] for eight years she was very interested in having me be with the four because of the heart energy that he taught. I didn't know that at the time but I found out later.

So, after back and forth and many discussions, we agreed to meditate once a week. I don't think it had to be the same time as the other three women, but we each did the same meditation on asking for guidance on taking the program out into the world instead of just keeping it in Colorado. It was a real commitment because this was before email, so every week we would mail letters out to each other. I'm not sure how long we did that, maybe a year, then we would see each other a couple of times a year at the holistic nurses conferences.

After we put the Healing Touch Program™ together, Janet asked the American Holistic Nurses Association (AHNA) to sponsor it. They wanted two pilot programs, one of which was done in Memphis, Tennessee and another in Florida. The program was approved as a certificate program and our first official Healing Touch conference was in Ft. Wayne, Indiana. Since I was on the holistic nurses board and had a mailing list of ten states, we had twenty-five people come.

That's how it got started, and then it just kind of evolved. Janet was our only instructor at the beginning, and I think she taught about twenty-five classes that first year. To become a certified instructor we had to go through all five levels of the program and to work alongside Janet for an unspecified number of classes. It was a real commitment for me because we lived over a thousand miles apart and I had to go to where she was in Colorado. When she thought we were ready to teach we would teach a Level I class. As the program continued to grow we got more and more instructors and the training to become an instructor became more rigorous. Part of the training was to observe a certain number of classes and co-teach a certain number, so the requirements gradually evolved into what they are today.

Since your book is about using energy healing at end of life I will share my experiences with you. I graduated from nursing school in 1957, and when we were seniors we were in charge of a floor at the hospital, working many nights and weekends. It seemed like on many of those nights I had patients who died. I always thought it was a privilege to be with someone as they were dying; even as a young student I was not afraid of it.

I remember one case in particular. It was Christmas Eve when my patient, a twelve-year-old boy, was dying from an accident. This was before intensive care units, so they put me in his room as a special-duty nurse to do what I could. I thought, "What am I doing here? I'm a student nurse and I'm in charge?"

He lived only a few hours and I'll always remember the parents coming up to me and thanking me, it's Christmas Eve, their son had just died, and they're thanking me. I will never forget this, their thanking me for being there with him. I didn't know anything about energy healing then, but I believe that being there for them and with them really helped, that sometimes just your presence makes a difference.

The other story that I want to tell you about, that says so much about presence, is about my grandson who died when he was 3½ years old. He had Tay-Sachs disease, a genetic disease that babies are born with. This disease used to be just within the Jewish culture, but there have been so many intermarriages that it's not limited to any particular culture any more. Both parents have to be carriers, with an A chromosome missing, and there is no cure for it.[2]

My grandson was like a normal baby until he was about eight or nine months old when he was diagnosed with the disease. At about five or six months it seemed he had gained a lot of weight and I wondered what had happened. Then I noticed at about eight months we would sit him on the couch and he would just kind of sit there and I thought, "This isn't right." I thought maybe he had brain damage or something but at about eight months he was diagnosed with Tay-Sachs disease. Soon he would just lie there, then he went blind, and then the seizures started. They became more frequent and lasted longer, sometimes as long as forty to forty-five minutes: that's a long time. This was before Healing Touch, but I had studied with Brugh Joy and I knew enough about the energy to modulate it. It's hard to do a chakra connection in a little kid, so I just did more of the modulating and the magnetic clearing techniques. Most of the time when I did that he would move out of the seizure within a minute.

Then the symptoms changed; he had a lot of respiratory problems, a cough, and needed to be aspirated with a machine. It was just ongoing constant care. I lived close by so I would get calls saying "I think he's dying, get over here." It was the seizures that would go on and on.

I tell people that my grandson was one of my greatest teachers even though he never said a word. I learned that when I got an emergency call and went over there, no matter what I did the seizures would continue as long as I was caught in my own emotional turmoil. Once I could calm down, and ground, and center my energy, the seizures would stop within a minute. So he really taught me how important it is to center and get one's emotions under control.

The other thing he taught me was healing versus curing. The medical model wants to cure everybody, and as a nurse I had helped a lot of people, so why couldn't I cure my own grandson? When I finally accepted that he wasn't going to be cured, but I could give him a quality of life while he lived, then I could move on and accept that. But it took a while to get to that point where I was able to see the difference. It was a valuable lesson when I first started energy work because as a nurse you are so geared to healing and curing everybody. We weren't taught to heal on the emotional level or mental or spiritual level.

My grandson died at our house on Christmas Eve. My son called and said that he was really bad, but he had been really bad for so long. My son and his wife went to Mass and while they were gone my husband and I just sat there and held and held him, we didn't say anything. When his parents came back his mother was dressing him, he took a breath, and he died in her arms. Only the four of us were there; my husband and myself, my son and his wife. I think it was very appropriate because we were the four who were the closest to him. Other family members were called and they stayed with us for a long time that night, they didn't want to leave. Finally they were able to let him go and the funeral director took him away. It was a very peaceful death with me doing the same things as always, the soothing, gentle passes with my hands and just holding him and directing heart energy to him.

For two years before he died I would be driving down the street, not thinking about him at all, and I would hear this voice inside saying, "You will speak at Joshua's funeral. You will." The first time I heard it, and it happened several times over those two years I said, "You're crazy." Here I am, talking to myself in the car. So I told the priest, "This is what I've been told, you may think I'm crazy, and I can't do it." He said, "I'll just announce at the end of the service if anybody wants to speak, you don't have to."

But when Mass started I felt a vibration in my body, I could just feel this revving up inside myself, I felt like my whole body was shaking but on the outside it wasn't moving. When the priest asked if anyone wanted to speak I felt two hands on my back, I felt these two hands, I felt myself stand up, I went to the front of the church and I started talking. When I started to speak there was a calmness that came over me.

I talked probably ten minutes and all I did was tell his life because he could never talk for himself. I remember saying that there were days I was angry with him for putting his parents through everything they were going through, and everybody in the church kind of gasped, like how can you be angry at a child? I found out that it was necessary to say the things that I did because nobody wanted to talk about his death, nobody wanted to talk about him because he died, he was a child, and we always wonder why God would do this to a child. I heard that many, many times, and I think just by telling the story of his life and how it affected all of us, I think that people understood a little bit more. Telling his story helped me. My sister asked me how long I had prepared for that talk and I laughed and said that I hadn't, it just flowed, it came from a different place.

After his death I felt a real void because I had worked with him so much, as did his parents. They were divorced within six months of his death; their whole focus had been on this child for three years.

I haven't worked a great deal with dying patients so there are not many stories to share, but there are two more that may interest you. The first is of a young man, about 19 or 20 years old, who came to me for energy healing when his cancer, which had been in remission, came back. When he left the session he looked so good, walked out like any other teenager, but I woke at 2:00 the next morning and I saw his face and he said "Thank You." That's the moment that he died. It was a shock to see him, it wasn't a dream, and a shock that he had died because he had looked so good just hours earlier.

The other story is about a family member who had uterine cancer. In February the cancer went into remission, but in April she started having pain and they found that the cancer had spread throughout her entire body. I had offered her Healing Touch and at first she had refused, but one Saturday she said yes, come on over. After the treatment she said that she felt so good that she was going to pull out her IV and I said, no, don't do that.

The following day was Mother's Day, and on Monday she went to the school her seven and nine-year-old children attended and was able to see them get some sort of award they had earned. On Wednesday she woke up and was really bad and she died that night. I look at the energy work as giving her a couple of days to be with her children, watch them get their awards, and then the rapid change and her death. The inevitable had happened, but I've always felt that the energy work had helped her, gave her some valuable time with her family.

So that is how doing energy healing has helped others, and now I will tell you how it has affected my life, both personally and professionally.

I had always wanted to change and grow holistically, had always been seeking holistic ways; that was just part of me. When I first met

Brugh Joy in 1980 and began to study with him this whole thing about energy was very foreign to me, I didn't know anything about it. I was not in a good marriage at the time and my interest in energy work just made it worse because now I was considered weird and strange.

I was supervising school nurses at the time and at our staff meetings we began to talk about what I was learning. Our nurses came together once a month and the whole afternoon they complained about this, they complained about that, and I kept thinking, "We've got to do something different here." I started taking them through a brief centering before the meeting, I would play a little music, and I look back now and half of them were probably thinking, 'Oh my god, what's she doing now?' and the other half really liked it; three or four of them went on to take the Healing Touch training when it came along. But it really changed our staff meetings, so I think I was brave enough to try something new. Often I thought I was going to be fired from my job if they heard me talk about this, because I gave some talks to the public, but it never happened.

So it helped me come out and talk more about who I was. I mean, it changed the whole direction of my nursing career, too, because at that time I was working full time, maybe teaching two weekends a month, sometimes three, it was just way too much, I never had a day off doing it that way.

One day I was at a meeting at the hospital that I graduated from and all of a sudden I felt this pressure in my chest. It went on for awhile and finally I said something to one of the nurses, that it was really bothering me. I didn't have any pain down my arm or any other symptoms but she thought I should go to the emergency room. As I was walking into the emergency room I heard something say: "It's okay if you go; you've done really well but if you choose to stay you need to recommit to your life." Recommit to what I didn't know, but that was the message.

They put me in the cardiac care unit that night, the EKG was irregular, and I thought, "This is a cosmic joke – why am I in the cardiac care unit, I teach heart stuff all the time, what am I doing here?" I was kind of mad that I had to be there, but of course it's not good to be mad at your heart, that's not good.

Even though I loved my job and knew I would miss the nurses, I made a decision about when I would quit and no longer do traditional nursing. I started teaching more Healing Touch, then I started seeing people and advertising, so my life evolved that way. I think my family certainly did not understand it, and my husband at that time didn't understand it at all. He thought all these weird people had changed my life, he just did not get it, and it *has* changed my life in a really good direction. I look back, and if I hadn't said yes to being on the Board when I was asked, and met Janet and the other people in the Healing Touch Program™, my life would have been different. My book is titled "Yes I Will," and I think about how saying yes changed my life in directions I would never have believed.

The Healing Touch training emphasizes self-care, so I do water aerobics every day, I meditate, I work on my dreams, I get massages, and I see a chiropractor about once a month when I need an adjustment to my neck. I see so many health care professionals who don't eat right, who don't exercise, who don't take care of themselves. I think health care professionals are the worst at taking care of themselves.

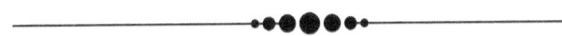

You asked me what I would like to tell people about death. Well, I believe that when we die we will continue to grow; when we leave this earth we're not just going to die and be happy and go to heaven in an afterlife like we were taught. It didn't make sense to me just to die, what do you do for eternity? For me I see it as a progression, so I feel the more we can grow here and accomplish our purpose the less work we have to do when we die; it's a transition.

Of course I've thought about death a lot because I'm older, and I don't think there's anything to fear, and yet there are times that I wonder how I'm going to die, things like that, what am I going to have to go through. I really believe that to take care of ourselves and to grow here while we still have a body is very important. I said to my son, "Right now in this time in my life is when I want to grow more spiritual. I don't mean church and religion, I mean to continue to expand my awareness and grow and teach as many people about living from the heart that I can." I said that jobs and all that aren't that important to me anymore as much as doing energy work and helping people.

Death, it's just continuing but without a body. My brother, the doctor, doesn't believe in life after death, he doesn't believe in God, he just believes when you die you die. No one really knows about death, and no one comes back to tell us, and I've heard that heaven is what you believe it is. I have had a few friends, though, who have had near-death experiences and they don't want to come back; it's a real letdown when they experience such a loving feeling like that. But it's always intrigued me when people die in plane crashes, or die suddenly as a group, what happens to them? They are here one minute and then they're gone; what happens to them? Are they confused? I think they are.

When a person is dying or in a coma, I believe you should talk to the person as if they are alive, as if they are there, alert, and can hear you. We've always been taught that hearing is the last to go, and I don't think people should stand in the room and talk about their work, and talk about everything else, and here you are, dying in the bed, and nobody is talking to you. I have seen, over and over again, when the family is in the room they don't die, and then the family goes to lunch or something and then they go. If you look at that energetically, the family is hanging on and they can't let go because the family wants them to stay.

One time I went to the hospital to do some energy work on the cousin of one of my friends. She was hooked up to all these monitors and my friend was saying, "Come on, you have to hang on, you have seven kids at home," and every time she said that you could see the blood pressure shoot up, you could see the respiration change, kind of bells went off because it was like she was screaming, "No, I can't!" The last time I saw my friend we talked about that, how all the monitors changed when she said that. The person died, but I just felt that fear.

When my mom died I was in the hospital with her all night and I just talked to her. She had a brain tumor and would have seizures, but I would just keep talking to her. I didn't know energy work at the time, that was 1978, but I believe in the presence, the healing presence. Now

I have Healing Touch which is wonderful in helping people ease into a very natural process.

Getting energy work into mainstream medicine remains a challenge but hospice has made a big difference. Most of the hospice programs that I know of have volunteers coming and they see and accept that Healing Touch helps with the pain, easing their patients into the dying process. There are a lot more people talking about energy work and there are a lot more programs than when I started in 1980. I was called a witch, devil, doing the devil's work, things like that. I think the consciousness has been raised, that it's more accepted now. We have seen the evolution of people's thinking about massages because it used to be that people thought only prostitutes gave massages, and that has totally changed. Acupuncture is more integrated but it takes somebody in the hospital or in the organization to really promote the complementary and alternative practices, it's hard to do when you're on the outside, not working at that place. So there is a shift, but it's not fast enough for me.

---

* Mary is a pseudonym. The name has been changed to protect the identity of family members mentioned in the interview.
1. W. Brugh Joy, MD, (1939-2009). Best known for his book Joy's Way: A Map for the Transformational Journey and for his workshops on the transformation of consciousness.
2. Tay-Sachs disease is a mutation of a gene known as the HEXA gene which regulates production of the hexosaminidase A enzyme. It progressively destroys nerve cells in the brain and spinal cord.

Debbie
Registered Nurse
Certified Clinical Aromatherapist
Healing Touch Certified Practitioner

Introduction

At the time of the interview Debbie had recently left hospice nursing to be a home health nurse, and before being a hospice nurse she had worked in a doctor's office where she introduced Healing Touch to the physician and the patients. Here is Debbie's story, beginning with my question to her, "What made you choose nursing as your profession?"

Interview

As a teenager I really didn't know what I wanted to do with my life and my mom suggested that I become a nurse. She only ever pushed me to do a couple of things, and that was one of them. She must have seen something in me that made her feel that I would be good at it, so I went to nursing school when I was eighteen. I really fell in love with the profession, and I just really love to help people to feel better, that you can improve whatever situation they're in.

After many years of traditional nursing, though, I was kind of getting burned out on it. My sister is a nurse in Washington state and she said, "Hey, I'm going to a Healing Touch class, a three-day class, it's the first level, fly up and we'll have a sister's weekend and we'll do this class together." That's how I was introduced to Healing Touch.

The first night I thought, "This just looks like voodoo," and then the next day when we started practicing I thought, "Oh, there is something to this," so then I just became very interested in it as a nurse. The more classes I went to I decided I wanted to become certified, that being certified would look better to hospitals, to doctors, that it would get me in the door if I were certified.

At first I was very embarrassed, very reluctant to use it. I mostly used it on friends and family and gradually gained confidence over the years. The surgeon I was working for paid for all the classes I was taking, which was nice, because I could get continuing education credits for nursing. So yes, it took me a lot of years to get confidence, to talk to doctors about it, to do it in the hospital or public settings, and now I could do it anywhere and I wouldn't care what anybody thought.

When I was first doing energy healing I would mostly just send people some energy while getting an injection, so it wasn't obvious. But the surgeon I was working for was very open to acupuncture, Ti Chi, yoga, all different types of modalities for treatment, so I presented him with the idea that anybody who was going to have spine surgery, that I offer Healing Touch to them pre-and post-op. That's where I think I got really comfortable doing it and talking to patients about it. We even had a flyer that went into their surgical packet, so I got very comfortable doing it and going to the hospital after a surgery and doing it on the patients. Patients who read about it in the pre-surgical packet, or patients I talked to in the office would contact me if they were interested. If they wanted to receive Healing Touch I would have them come to my office a day or two before surgery and I would do a pre-op treatment. Then, after they had their surgery I would go over to the hospital. Sometimes I would see them several times after their surgery if they had extensive back surgery.

The feedback I got from patients was very positive, especially when I was working directly over their spine to accelerate healing and to clear out the anesthetics. The hospital staff were really receptive, too. They were starting to teach the basics of Healing Touch in the nursing program at the local university, so a lot of the nurses had an awareness of it although in the hospital we have to refer to it as comfort touch. They were very open to me going into a patient's room, and I would put a sign on the door saying, "Comfort touch in session. Please do not disturb if at all possible." They were actually kind of relieved because I was in there taking care of the patient for them so they could do something else.

I think the surgeon that I worked for became a believer in Healing Touch when he witnessed what happened to one of his patients. The patient was so sedated, his pain had been so out of control after the surgery, that they could hardly wake him up. I did an hour-long Healing Touch treatment on him in the morning and when the doctor did his rounds later that day he came back to the office and said, "He's a different person." And it was true, you could just see this huge difference in him; he was awake, not having a lot of pain.

———————————— •••●●●•• ————————————

After I left that job I worked as a hospice nurse for seven years. There were a couple of different categories of patients I would see. Some people would just have me come see them when they were very close to death as a way to control agitation that no medications could subdue, so those patients I would just see once or twice. That would be the calmest time for them, during Healing Touch and the few hours afterwards.

There were some patients that I would see every single week until they died, and that sometimes went on for months or years. One patient who was on home hospice care I saw once a week for two years, so some of the patients I got a really close relationship with. I would show up to do Healing Touch for anxiety, on another day it might be pain, it would vary, but I would really get to know them. When they got close to death we already had this established relationship, and it was very comforting for them to already know me so well and for me to help them through the final phase.

I would sometimes teach family members to do some of the techniques, but since I was on nursing assignment and had time constraints there wasn't much time to teach. On average I would spend forty-five minutes doing a Healing Touch treatment but it was very individual. I would always ask them how long they wanted me to work on them and some would want only thirty minutes, some would want an hour, and some would want it all day long if they could get it.

Family members benefited, also. I saw one of my patients for five or six months and then I started doing sessions with his wife, as well. Then their dog got sick so I gave the dog a treatment using the techniques I had learned in Healing Touch for Animals, so everybody's chakras were open by the time I left.

Whenever I saw a patient, especially at their home, whoever was in the room got the benefit of the treatment. Sometimes I would have the spouse lie down on the other side of the bed if it was a normal bed while everything was happening, or there would be a dog on the floor, so even though I wasn't doing Healing Touch on the spouse the music, the oils, the energy in the room would be very calming and relaxing. If I had time I would do a brief intervention on the other person, as well as the patient, and usually I would put everybody to sleep. I would tell them ahead of time, "Frequently, people fall asleep. If that happens I'm not going to wake you up to say goodbye, I'm just going to tip-toe out very quietly." The chaplains hated coming after me, they would say, "Debbie, we never want to follow you because everybody's asleep."

There are particular Healing Touch interventions that I use depending upon what the goal is, which could be pain relief, stress and anxiety reduction, calm their agitation, and/or relieve nausea. We are taught in the program to use the chakra spread when people are going through major transitions, including the transition from life into death. I used it on my mom a lot when she was dying and she always said it felt so good.

There was one lady who actually died during the chakra spread, and that was very interesting. I had only met her once before, and I showed up at the nursing home to do it and three of her five children were in the room. She was Catholic, and she had some Catholic hymns being played. The Catholics are really into frankincense, so I made sure that I put frankincense and two other biblical oils, I think it was the cedar wood and the cypress on her, and I was almost done with the chakra spread when one of her kids goes, "I don't think she's taken another breath." It was so beautiful, so peaceful.

So I stopped, and they all just kind of held her, and we talked for a little bit, and we listened to the music; it was beautiful. The kids were so grateful that they were there, that I was there doing that when she passed, the oils, the Healing Touch, the music. They were so impressed that when their father, who had dementia, was dying a year or so later, they called our office to ask if a Healing Touch practitioner could come out. He wasn't even a hospice patient but the experience they had with their mother and me had impressed them so much that they wanted the same for their father. They even wrote down the names of the oils I used, it was very important to them, because they wanted to share it with their other siblings.

Some of the oils, particularly the calming oils, I would put on the soles of the feet, just rub a little in. For nausea I might rub a little peppermint on their belly or on the stomach reflex point on their feet, and I might also put a little lavender on their feet because lavender is calming. Some oils I might just put a slight smear across their forehead, or a little bit on a cotton ball so the aroma is released into the room. I think it's important to study the oils and the reflexology points in order to use oils therapeutically. My experience is that using oils and Healing Touch in combination complements each other and makes them more powerful.

When giving a treatment I always use music; I almost can't do it without music. Sometimes I use something from my collection but I ask my patients if they have a particular kind of music that they want. I remember one patient who really liked Indian drums and flute, so I went out and bought a tape of that. Tammy Briggs is a harpist and music therapist and I use a lot of her music. For some patients I use CDs of calming music, and for the patients who love hymns I play those. I had a CD of harp music that was just all the old hymns and it was a favorite of a lot of my older patients. Healing Touch, essential oils, music; it's kind of like being in heaven before you go, it's a perfect combination.

In hospice we had a lot of COPD patients. With COPD (chronic obstructive pulmonary disorder) a person has trouble breathing, shortness of breath, and I found that the combination of Healing Touch, essential oils, and music worked really well with them. Their respirations would be very rapid, but by the end of a Healing Touch session their breathing was very relaxed, they were dozing, so they had gone from a state of anxiety and difficulty breathing to their breathing being relaxed and the anxiety gone.

Some of the ladies I saw didn't have anxiety, they didn't have pain, but they loved the pampering of Healing Touch. Everyone else was showing up to do other things, but I was just there to pamper them. I would throw in some hand and foot massage with the Healing Touch, so they kind of felt like I was their masseuse, they were going to the spa, or I was bringing the spa to them. There were a couple of ladies that I would see every week and it was the highlight of their week. They would kick their families out, tell them to go away, be quiet, this is my time.

Everybody had different needs and wants from the Healing Touch, there were all these different categories: people with severe agitation, people in pain, and people who just wanted to be pampered. I had one patient, a man whom I knew only for one week before he died, who called my boss and asked if I could come out every day. The normal schedule is to see a patient once a week, but I went out three times that last week of his life and he loved it.

There are so many stories I could tell you. Richard was one of my COPD patients whom I saw once or twice a week for two years. He didn't really think there was anything to this Healing Touch when he was first told about it, but as time went on he realized the value of it. I would show up and he would be having back pain and I would work on that, his breathing would be bad, or he would just have some anxiety, so he really changed from a non-believer into a believer. It was interesting to see how he came around to being a believer and finding such value in it.

We developed a deep friendship; I would sometimes bring him meals, I would take leftovers or I would bake brownies for him, whatever. I wasn't with him at the time of his death, I had seen him just a couple of days before he passed, but I was with him on his journey most of the way. I still miss him, but he had gotten so miserable. A lot of patients I really got attached to because I saw them for so long, but they got so miserable at the end that I would actually be asking for a peaceful passing, it was just time to transition.

There was another patient, a woman that I saw for several months. She was young, only in her late 30s, and she was dying of cancer. She was really open to my Healing Touch and oils for awhile, and then she just abruptly didn't want me to come out for about a month. Then she decided that I could come back out and she told me that the reason she hadn't wanted to see me was because the energy healing was bringing a lot of emotional issues to the surface that she really didn't want to deal with; it just brought too much emotional stuff to the surface. We know that is a good thing, but she needed a break from that for awhile before she was ready to continue. She was a hard one for me because she was so young and had young children.

Another category of people I saw were the ones with dementia and Alzheimer's but I always wondered how much I impacted them. I had seen one lady for a couple of months with pretty significant dementia and most of the time she just talked nonsensical, her answers made no sense. One day I was leaving and she just looked at me with this clarity and said, "Thank you." That felt so good because she never talked that way. You just never know how much impact you have on those types of patients, you just have to let go of an outcome, but I think it really helps. I just looked at her and said, "Thank you for saying that." It was so sweet.

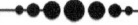

Being a Healing Touch practitioner has impacted me both personally and professionally. On a personal level it has really motivated me to meditate every morning and to do good self-care because you can't do energy work if you're tired and not taking care of yourself, you're not grounded. When I was younger I didn't do very good self-care, so it has taught me to take great care of myself and to take that time in the morning before I leave the house to pray and to meditate.

I've worked on most of my family members and friends for various things, including post-surgery for pain and accelerated healing. My granddaughter is very interested in what I do. She likes to check the chakras to see what is happening with them, and if she doesn't feel good she will say, "I need an oil, Grandma."

Professionally it taught me that in the traditional medical world there is more than one modality that you can use. I love combining traditional medicine with alternative medicine, having that integrative medicine; to me, that is the best of both worlds in almost any situation.

I was definitely burned out on traditional nursing: I was bored, I was burned out, I needed something different.

You mentioned that many of the nurses that you have interviewed said that they were getting burned out, that nursing was not the healing profession that they wanted it to be, but when they found Healing Touch or other similar energy healing modalities they really felt they were back aligned with their original intention of being a healer. I have to agree with that. A lot of times there is only so much you can do for a patient, and I always wish I could do something more to make them feel better, so to be able to pull out these other tools is awesome.

When I first became a nurse, that was in 1979, I worked swing shift and every patient got a back rub at bedtime. We had that human touch of just doing that calming thing of rubbing somebody's back before they went to sleep for the night. So Healing Touch kind of brings back that old basic of nursing, that human touch. There is so much of the mechanical and electronic going on now, especially with hospital patients, they don't really get touched. Aides are even trained to wear gloves to put lotion on them.

Some people don't want to be touched or to receive Healing Touch, which is fine because it can be done without ever touching the body. Some people have a religious objection to any type of healing they don't consider directly from God, and some just don't like touch. I had a couple of people in hospice where I gave them only one treatment and they never wanted me to come back again. They were older women who had never liked being physically touched their entire lives. Of course I honor their wishes.

What I want people to know is that it's just another modality, another treatment that, if they can open their minds to it may benefit them more than they can imagine and how it can complement any treatment that they are already doing, whether it's traditional medicine, surgery, or whatever the case may be. You can add it to anything and it's just going to complement, it's not going to take away from whatever other treatments they are doing.

Since I've had a lot of experience with death, I'll share my perspective with you. I think that death is similar to the birth of a baby, they're both a transition, they're both a sacred time, they're very special. They are on different ends of the spectrum, but I think they both can be just as joyous and special and spiritual and sacred. If you can be at a birth, it's very special, and if you can be with somebody when they take their last breath, that can be very special. I was with my mom when she took her last breath, and it was very, very special.

I realized that she was probably going to die in a couple of weeks because she had had a spinal stroke, and I knew she wasn't going to be able to eat or drink, so I asked her, "Is there anything you're afraid of with death?" And she said, "The only thing I'm afraid of is that you won't be there with me when it happens."

I saw her one evening and the next morning I just knew I needed to go see her again, so I let them know at work I wouldn't be there. Mom had become totally unresponsive and I knew she was going to die that day. I stayed with her, did Healing Touch, repositioned her, did nursing stuff, and just prayed that it would go quickly. Right before she took her last breath she actually opened her eyes, with a look of awe, like she was seeing to the other side, thinking something like "This is better than I imagined." I just said, "Mom, go to heaven," and she took one last breath and she died. It was just peaceful and I was there like she wanted me to be. It was very sacred. That was so special. I'm very glad I got that intuitive message to go see her that morning.

When people fear death I think they fear the unknown. There are a couple of categories I've seen; people with unfinished business, and people with spiritual anxiety. If a person still has a lot of what I would call emotional garbage it seems it's very hard for them to leave this life because there are so many things they haven't taken care of; people they still hate, unresolved relationships, regrets. People who have emotionally taken care of things and moved on seem happier and they don't have the agitation and anxiety like the others do. And then spiritually, if you know where you're going that takes away a lot of the fear. But no matter what it can be somewhat fearful because it's an unknown journey, but I think the more people are emotionally healthy and happy the less the fear, and the less the anxiety and the agitation. I tell everybody, just communicate, take care of things, forgive.

Is there such a thing as a good death or a bad death? The people who seem to have the peaceful death are just emotionally balanced. They usually believe in God, they believe in an afterlife, they believe in heaven, so they're not fearful of where they're going. They've taken care of things, they have all their emotional and spiritual things in order. And then there are people who, maybe it's the kind of life they've led, maybe they've done some really bad things, or they don't believe in an afterlife, I think they don't know where they're going and they're terrified, just terrified. I've been with those people and it's just awful to see what they're going through. They're tossing and turning and trying to get out of bed, they're restless, they're agitated, they're yelling and screaming, they're combative; it's extremely hard to calm them down and just kind of surrender. In cases like that we give them pharmaceuticals, do Healing Touch, the oils, the music, but in those really agitated deaths everything helps but nothing takes away all of it.

Most people see a little light, but there was one lady whose caretaker told me that the patient was seeing the gates of hell in her bedroom and she was terrified and agitated. She was screaming and yelling and finally, I guess, in the middle of the night she finally said, "Okay, God, I choose you," and although she said it in an angry tone of voice, from that point on she calmed down and died peacefully several hours later.

Many people die in the middle of the night when it's quiet. My personal belief, and that of other hospice nurses, is because it's a very spiritual, private experience and they want to die when there aren't a bunch of people around them. I think that sometimes the energy of family and friends can hold them back if they don't want the person to go. I've had a lot of family members who feel so guilty that they weren't with their loved one for that last breath and I tell them, "You know what? A lot of people want to be alone, and that's why they die at 2:00 in the morning, or when everybody is out of the room. They want it quiet, they don't want anybody around, it's a private, spiritual journey and they are disconnecting from everything in this life, so don't feel guilty." I often warn people that this may happen. It's important to ask your loved one what they want before it's too late and they can't talk any more. If you are one of the people who doesn't want to die alone it's important that you tell your family so they know your wishes.

Families of patients that I have worked with for a long time tell me how important it is to them when I can be there at the time of death, someone they like and trust. It's meaningful for me, too; it's intimate, it's sacred, it's spiritual. But sometimes it's an animal that is with the person at the end. In a lot of the assisted care centers that I went to they'll have resident cats or dogs and the cats, especially, like to go lie on the person's bed who is the sickest or is starting to die. There have been many stories that the cat actually would go to the next person who was going to die. I think we don't give animals enough credit. I think they're intuitive, they have emotions, they sense things, they like to help heal, they like to comfort. I had one patient who had died and his dog was spooning him in bed in the hospital.

They give, but they like to receive, too. One of my cats would be in the room every time I gave a treatment if I let her. She likes to lie on a person's legs or somewhere in the middle of their body. Maybe that's their way of giving and receiving at the same time, just like we humans do in our healing work.

Elaine
Hospice Chaplain

Introduction

Debbie, whose interview you just read, suggested several people whom she thought would be interested in sharing their experiences with Healing Touch and one of those was Elaine, the wife of one of Debbie's patients who received home hospice care. Elaine is not a practitioner but saw and personally experienced the benefits of the energy healing that her husband received. After her husband's death Elaine went on to become a hospice chaplain.

Interview

I met Debbie when my husband was receiving home care nursing for pulmonary fibrosis. His Veterans Administration (VA) lung specialist said that he had no doubt that it was primarily caused from Agent Orange while he was a soldier in Viet Nam. He was a gunner on a helicopter for awhile, a mechanic on all the trucks and other vehicles, and was just in among all the foliage a lot of the time.

The VA doctor told my husband that he needed to be on hospice, so he was on hospice for about a year before he took himself off. We were going to Mexico for treatments once a year to get stem cell shots, and the first two years it really helped him a lot. He was able to breathe much easier, not use nearly as much oxygen, so he felt he was doing well and didn't need hospice. After the third trip my husband said it just wasn't doing much for him any more and he wasn't planning to go back.

We were still seeing his doctor at the VA during this time and he told my husband he thought he should go back on hospice. They started sending Debbie out once a month to do Healing Touch and she and Don got to be really good friends. Don just thought she was a wonderful lady, and I thought she was, too, because when she was there with Don it helped me so much. As soon as she would get there and turn her music on I would say "Bye," and would head for my bedroom because I knew that was the one time during the month that I could just get away and totally not worry about Don. I knew he was in good hands, that he was getting what he needed and I could relax, go back to my bedroom, lay down, if I wanted to go to sleep I could sleep and know that he was in perfectly good hands. Or if I just needed to go lay down and relax and rest, just close my mind to everything else, I knew as long as Debbie was working on Don I had no fear of him not being in perfect hands and I didn't have to worry. I didn't have to be listening for the oxygen, I didn't have to be watching him to see if his pain level was where we needed to get some morphine in him, I knew that it was a time I could just go away, somewhere far away, and be okay with that.

So yeah, when Debbie would come out to see Don it was a great relief for him, she could just make him totally relax and he would feel so much more rested and relaxed because of the treatment. It was a very restful, peaceful time for both of us while Debbie was there. I could see the anxiety just leave him; he would be just peaceful and at rest. That anxiety, a lot of the pain was gone for several hours, so it just put him in a really good place mentally and physically.

Don was good at hiding what he was going through from other people, but when you've lived with someone for forty years you know when they're hiding their emotions and their pain. So, to walk back into the room after Debbie was finished, and to see that relaxed state that he was in, I mean to the point where he would just drift off to sleep and sleep for a long time. His sleep pattern was just really bad, but after Debbie would finish with him I could just see the peace. He could just sit there in his recliner and really relax and be at peace with everything.

When your loved one suffers you suffer, too. It's so devastating to not be able to do anything for somebody that you love. As a hospice chaplain I feel that way about my patients, the desire to help relieve their suffering, I just want to do something for them. So when I see the peace that my patients are in after they have received comfort touch, and the lack of pain on their faces, even for just a short time, it means so much to me because I know, personally, what relief they've gotten.

After my husband died I started volunteering at the agency where Debbie worked because I wanted to give something back to them for being so wonderful with helping him. I started just as a volunteer in the office and I was also going to a grief support group. Being a part of that, I learned that I could help other people with their losses, so again, just as a volunteer, I started helping with the grief support groups.

At first I was reluctant to go to a grief support group because I already had a strong support group in my two church communities and my family. The facilitator kept inviting me to attend her group and I finally said yes just to get her off my back. Well, I stayed for about three years and every time I thought "Okay, that's it, I won't be back," somebody new would come in and we would have a connection to where I was helping them in their grief so I never got a chance to leave. The connections with the people and the facilitators helped me get through my grief.

I discovered that the group was different than my other support systems. In group that's what we were there for, to talk about our loss. If we needed to sit there through the whole hour or hour and a half and cry it was okay, there was nobody there that you felt was thinking "Won't you just shut it up and get on with it? Aren't you over it by now? I'm uncomfortable, I don't want to see you crying." You just knew that your tears were okay, whatever you said about your grief and your feelings was okay, nobody was judging you. As other people talked about their grief and their emotions you are like, "Oh, I guess I'm not crazy, there are other people feeling that same exact thing." So it just really helps so much to be able to talk with people you know are going through that same emotion, that same hurt, and to just know that you're not the only person in the world feeling like that.

As a society it's like, "Okay, you've got a week and you've got to be over it and back on your feet and going at it again. And don't make us feel uncomfortable by letting us see tears and emotions because that's just not where we want to be." So when you can share that with other people and everybody is having those same emotional ups and downs, and you know other people are hurting as bad as you are, it is very healing.

It was wonderful, I loved it, but I kept feeling like there was something more that I needed to be doing. So I just kept praying, "Lord, I know there's something more for me, but you're going to have to show me." I kept praying, "Lord, I really, really would like a job at the agency where I am, but where I could help more than I am now."

Before long I just kind of felt like He was telling me to be a chaplain and I argued back, "not me," but I kept getting that feeling over and over. So I thought, "okay," and I approached the head of the program who said they needed a woman chaplain part time, which was exactly what I wanted. When I was still questioning whether being a chaplain was the right thing to do I was lying in bed one night and I felt Don's hand on my back, just very lightly on my back, giving me a little shove, and I knew it was Don saying, "Yeah, this is what I want you to do, this is what you need to be doing."

That was one of the times I know for sure that he came to me after he died. Another time there were a pair of doves sitting, looking into the living room window and watching me as I moved around the room. For thirty years we had both enjoyed the doves on our property, nesting in the trees, sitting on the electrical and telephone wires, but they had never come to the house like this before. I knew that was a sign from Don, that he was just fine, that everything was good.

After Don died I felt like there was no reason for me to live, I actually thought about taking my life because what use was there for me? But if you stay strong in your faith, and you get with the right people that can help you through your grief, there is a reason to go on living, there's hope, there's purpose, *there is purpose in life* after you've lost your loved one. I think that's my greatest desire, to help people know that there is a reason to go on living, there's purpose. You're going to miss that loved one for the rest of your life but you can deal with it, and you can go on and find a reason to keep living and keep going.

When one of my patients is going through something really hard it is stressful for me but I just depend on the Lord so much. My minister is an amazing man and it's like his sermons, the Lord just gives him something that I can really take in and apply it to myself. This is part of my self-care, and it seems like when things have really been hard the Lord just kind of gives me time to myself or sends somebody along, like my sister, that I can just relax with and have a few laughs.

But death itself is not scary, it's actually a very peaceful thing. This sounds strange, I know, but it's a beautiful thing, and to be with people when they transition to the other side, it's like watching them go into a brilliant, bright, beautiful place. And to watch the pain being released, to see that they're not in pain any more, they're just at peace, so at peace.

I was told by one health care worker who came out to see my husband that at the very end of life, when they take that last breath, there are things about the body that are not real pleasant, but I haven't seen that at all. My husband died when I was away from the house and I was so scared to walk in the door because I remembered all of this horrible stuff I had been told would happen; I was so afraid to walk in and see my husband and what kind of condition he would be in. It wasn't that way, not at all. He was sitting in his recliner with his eyes closed and he looked very, very peaceful. He wasn't cold, I took his hand, and it was just like I was holding his hand any other time. He had not made a mess all over himself, it was just like walking in and seeing him so peacefully asleep, having a nap except there wasn't the pain on his face; it was like I was seeing him fifteen years ago.

So death is not a scary, nasty, messy thing. My patients, I haven't seen that, I just see them take a breath and they're gone, that pain has left them and they're just so peaceful. So I don't know who decided to give people this picture of death being scary and messy and icky, I don't know where that came from, because it's just not something that I have seen. Yes, you need to teach people about the end of life and about death, but I haven't seen what they said to expect. My experience is that it's not a scary thing, it's really a beautiful thing, and to be sitting with someone as they transition, it's a beautiful thing, it's a blessed time. There's definitely a different feeling in the room, it's like a feeling of peace. There's often a feeling of another presence there, it's not like I see anything, it's just the feeling of a peaceful presence.

I wasn't with my mom when she died, but I had been there for hours and hours and my sisters and my nephew had all been there, said our goodbyes and told her, "Mom, it's okay for you to go home and be with the Lord." There was a very definite presence in the room then, and it was just a few hours later that they called and said that she had passed. But I could see on my mother's face, I think she had transitioned before she took her last breaths. There was almost a glow around her and she kept looking out the window by her bed. I don't know if she even knew that the family was there, but she just kept looking out that window like she was expecting that window to take her away.

In the year that I've been a chaplain there is only one patient who I would say had a difficult death. This lady was in a lot of pain from cancer that wasn't able to be controlled by the drugs. We had talked before she became too far gone to be able to talk, she was definitely a believer and wanted to leave this world and go to heaven, so I don't know what was holding her back. I sat with her for quite some time, I prayed with her, but it felt as if there might be something that she was fighting. I didn't know her well enough to know if there might be something and if there was what that might be.

Easy, peaceful deaths seem to happen when people are ready to leave this world and go home and be with the Lord. Even if they're in pain, if they're ready and they know what's on the other side for them the transition is easy.

Ben
Bachelor of Arts
Masters in Divinity
Hospital Chaplain

Introduction

The next story is also about a chaplain, a hospital chaplain. When I contacted him for an interview he didn't think he was a good candidate since he had only completed Level I of the Healing Touch Program™ and didn't use energy healing regularly in his work, but I encouraged an interview anyway. As you will see from his story, a basic training in Level I techniques combined with a deep desire to relieve suffering can make a significant difference in people's lives.

Interview

As a hospital chaplain I assess and provide emotional and spiritual needs of patients and families. I found out about Healing Touch through an announcement of classes being offered in this area and decided to take the class. My awareness of healing and the ability to communicate at a level other than just the conscious level happened when I watched a program about an animal communicator on the animal channel. She said that we can train ourselves to be in tune with animals and with people and I thought that was wonderful. It would mean so much to me, to be able to be in tune with people, because people who are on ventilators in the hospital cannot talk, they are so distressed and in so much agony, and it seems to me they are saying, "Please help me."

But I felt pretty helpless with the vent (ventilator) dependent patients in the Intensive Care Unit (ICU). They cannot talk, some can communicate in writing, but most patients, having that tube in their throat is so uncomfortable. So here's a patient on a vent, some are heavily sedated and sleeping most of the time and the family are there, so there is nothing much that I can do for the patient. I can talk to the patient and the family, do whatever I can to be helpful to them, but for the patients I feel helpless. I say a prayer, that I can do, but is there something else that I can do?

I don't have the skill that the animal communicator has, and I wanted to help, so that is why energy healing sounded like it might be something I could use to help my patients. I want to help people find comfort and strength during their crisis, so now when I see a patient in distress I can offer them Healing Touch. After many years of helping patients you get the sense of knowing if a patient is in so much distress that the medicines cannot help. I will give you an example.

A lady had to have emergency surgery on her throat because of an acute infection. Because of the swelling after the surgery she wasn't able to breathe through her mouth or nose so she had to have a tracheostomy, a hole in the throat. She was really uncomfortable breathing through this hole; it caused congestion and a lot of severe headaches. She was allowed to take her medication only every four hours but she suffered in between times. I asked the nurse if she could get it sooner, "She is in so much pain," but I was told she had to wait another hour or so. I felt sorry for her, she was in so much distress, pain and agony, too much pain.

So I said to her, "If you want to, I'd like to offer you something that can help you. It's called Healing Touch, it can help you to relax, and when your mind relaxes your whole body opens up. You will have better circulation, your pain may reduce, it's totally up to you." That's how I do it, how I introduce it to patients. Sometimes very pleasant people will hide their anxiety so well, but by talking and probing a little bit I can find out if that patient has anxiety or worry. So then I offer Healing Touch when nothing else is available to help that person with their distress. That's how I got into this, interested in Healing Touch, because of my sense of helplessness in helping the people. So it was "Ah, here's something that I can do!"

So going back to the woman who had surgery on her throat, she said, "Yes, I'd like to try it." I explained to her, "I'm going to play nice music and I'm going to use techniques, some hands on, some hands off, is that okay with you?" She said yes, so I got permission from the nurse and told her I needed one hour without interruption.

The music that I use is very simple harp music, a very simple arrangement, so it's almost like a lullaby. Some people don't like the sound of the ocean or they are scared of it, so I just use this simple one, like twinkle, twinkle little star, memories of being an infant. I closed the door and did Healing Touch and within fifteen minutes she was sound asleep and snoring. I finished the session and went out without waking her up and a couple of hours later when I checked back she was awake and said, "I had a good power nap, thank you very much." The pain reduced, the congestion released, and it was a good outcome. So whenever I see patients whose distress is not being relieved by the medication, that's when I offer the Healing Touch. I tell them that we have volunteers available if you want but it's totally up to you. I tell them it can help you to relax and reduce the pain, and I say that my experience is that eight out of ten patients who receive this therapy fall asleep during the session and have a nice power nap. That's how I approach it.

People at first ask me what it is, what's Healing Touch? I tell them that it's a relaxation technique, it helps them to relax, you come in this way, tense, and when you're tense your blood pressure goes up, but with the Healing Touch your whole system is calmed and becomes still, that's the purpose of this therapy. Nobody has said no to me, but I give them the option to say no now or later if they have tried it and don't want any more.

Another of my patients that I think about was a prisoner who was on a vent. A young man, very agitated, a vent in the throat, a terrible, terrible thing for a young man to be in that situation. The prison guard was just sitting there, totally callous about his agony. So I asked, "Can I offer you something? This can help you to breathe better, to feel better," but before I did that I said, "You are labeled as a prisoner but here you are our patient who deserves care, our care, that we give to everybody else. You are a child of God, too, and to Him you are a precious person." As I do the energy healing I say a prayer as

41

I move up the body, starting at the ankles, on up to the knees and to every major joint in the body, and above the major organs. I repeat the prayer silently: "May this part of your body be at peace, free of stress, full of love and energy." As I take a deep breath in and out I breathe those positive energies into that part of the body. Then I move to the next part of the body and so on, so I breathe those positive energies of peace, health, strength, hope, love to every cell of their body. So that's how I do it, I pour my love into that patient.

Of course the patient doesn't know what I'm praying, I say the prayer silently, but before I start I tell them, "While I do this, move my hands to different parts of your body, I'm going to send you good energy by saying, 'May you be at peace in this moment, may your body become stronger,' and I'm going to repeat this as I move." That way the person knows my intention and he or she knows that my mind is here, not over there somewhere. This is what I did with the young man, I spent about ten minutes with him, fully present, and he fell asleep. That ability to help someone so profoundly was what I had been looking for.

I use some healing techniques that I've learned but I know that my intention, my care for that person, pure love for them will do more benefit than my techniques, so that's my focus. I learned something so precious from the instructor of a music healing program, it was so comforting and encouraging to me that it's not your technique, it's your intention that will bring healing to that person. The moment that you walk into the room of a patient your presence itself is healing. We're not here to show our ability, it's not a performance, it's a service. It's not about you, it's about them. Facial expression, tone of voice, everything; you set the mood.

Generally, the responses that I get are that the patients become so relaxed, like they are in the arms of their mother or their loved ones. I can see on the monitor that the elevated vital signs go down, their heart rate and everything. It is so cool to see that. At first the numbers are over there, as you get deeper into the therapy, five minutes, ten minutes, fifteen minutes, breathing, respiratory rate, heart rate, blood pressure, are all normalizing; it's amazing to see that. Most of them fall asleep. I am so happy that I can do that for the patients.

I haven't actually checked to see if the ventilator tube comes out sooner for patients whom I have done the Healing Touch on as compared to patients that I haven't, but the nurses notice something, so they say please come back and do this for my patients. Most of them in the ICU see the benefits. I have heard that the patients got out of the vent quicker through this kind of therapy, or music therapy, but in my personal experience I don't know since I may see the patient only the one time, but the ICU nurses can tell you.

I use Healing Touch for any patient who is anxious, not just those who are vent-dependant. One patient I saw was a woman in her 80s here to have brain surgery to get a hematoma evacuated. She was extremely anxious about the surgery. I had no idea what was going on in her mind except that she requested a chaplain. I offered a prayer and a Healing Touch technique that helps a person relax and experience a calmer mind. The surgery was successful and she was discharged to another facility for rehab.

One day her social worker called me, asking me to visit with her. She added that the patient found faith in God through my visit, which was a total surprise to me because we hadn't discussed her faith at all. When I visited her I was even more surprised when she said that she had been able to let go of her anger toward God who had not heard her prayers to save her two children 50 or 60 years ago. She said that during my pre-op visit with her, her anger and resentment of many years was lifted from her heart and that she found peace within herself and with God. What a surprise!

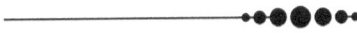

Before becoming a hospital chaplain I was a minister and I didn't know what I was getting into by changing professions. I thought it was the same thing, you pray for a patient to get well and sometime it works and sometimes it doesn't and then you feel helpless to be of help, like I did with the vent patients. Through the chaplaincy training we become comfortable, not a hundred percent, but we become comfortable dealing with the helpless situations. There are lots of helpless situations here: spinal cord injuries, head injuries, and what can you do? Some make a very slow recovery and just a little progress, others no progress at all, so what do you do? You've got to feel comfortable with that feeling of helplessness.

Actually, when you feel uncomfortable, when you feel the pain of that helplessness with that person, then that becomes a gift to them. When you are way up here (gestures with his hands up high) and they are down there (gesturing low), they don't feel that connection. When you can say "I feel that pain, too," that empathy, then you are connected with that person.

With pastors our training is to be a Messiah, to save people from their troubles, personal troubles, or marriage troubles or family problems, this and that, church problems, we save people, rescue people, like the Messiah. But that orientation doesn't work here so we have to change that mindset from trying to do something to being with that person, feeling the pain of the helplessness, hopelessness, feel the pain. That itself is a gift, you yourself are a gift. Not what you do for the person, but you yourself is a gift, feel the pain together. It was a difficult transition, but through the years we begin to see the value to that: I feel pain, and that's alright.

So, even though we have that training, how to deal with helplessness, still I want to help those helpless people, like the vent dependent people and I can do that through Healing Touch. Sometimes not only vent dependent patients, but other patients with chronic problems and so on, who are very distressed. Cancer drains a person's energy, so I ask, "Can I help you to regain your strength?" It's comforting that I can do something for them to recharge their energy.

It's difficult for family members to watch their loved ones suffering, so they feel so relieved when something can help them. There is so much comfort for them, it relieves their anxiety to see that something is working. Sometimes I offer that to the family, too, because they are so stressed out, so I ask, "Can I help you, too, to relieve your stress?" In our ICU rooms we have a nice lazy chair, a recliner, so I have them sit there, I put a small blanket over their body, and I usually just do one technique that is so relaxing that takes no longer than fifteen minutes.

I find being a hospital chaplain much more rewarding than being a church pastor. I still go to church, I still have my spiritual practices, and through the chaplaincy training we have to learn the spiritual practices of other religions. So now I'm incorporating practices from Buddhism, Islam, even shamanism.

The hospital here is so flexible, they allow me to try anything, so I don't just use Healing Touch, prayer, and music, I use line dancing also. One pediatric patient was so anxious about her surgery, so I called the two CNAs whom I trained in dancing in gangnam style and the three of us went in and were ready to dance for her. I said to her, "You must know gangnam style," and she said, "Yes!" "Do you want to join us?" So she got out of the bed, with the patient gown on, stood by our side and we started to dance. She became so happy that she ran to the OR with a smile.

After one surgery the baby was crying non-stop; Mom, Grandma, no one could calm her, just crying non-stop. The mom saw us line dancing so she came out of her room with her baby in her arms. The baby saw us dancing and she stopped crying. Even when we were finished dancing, no more crying! So whatever works, you know. Interesting that each thing has its own effect.

My main job as a chaplain is listening, but sometimes it takes awhile to get down to what is really going on with a patient, where the healing really needs to be. I was called to the ER one night at 11:30 pm. The house manager said that a patient came in with chest pain but he didn't have a heart problem, just the pain, so that is most likely anxiety-related pain. So I came into the hospital, read his chart, and I found him to be a walking hospital patient census, he's got everything: cancer, diabetes, hypertension, depression, there were so many things wrong with this man. The house manager said, "He is very afraid of death and dying." So I walked in and said, "I heard you are very afraid of death and dying," and instead of him answering his wife said, "Yeah, he's been fearful of death for many years." So I said, "Tell me about what is going on with you."

We talked for two hours and he shared the experience of his brother dying when they were young, which made him completely lose his faith in God, and later as a young man in Viet Nam he had had to call in a bombing mission, and on another occasion he killed an enemy soldier who shot at him. He had carried around the guilt of these deaths for forty years and felt that he deserved all the illnesses that he had. I was able to share a story of my own from many years back when I was in the mission field and a woman who was helping me went into a diabetic coma and died. I felt that my carelessness had caused her death, and I had been carrying that guilt and sorrow for many years.

While he was listening to my story he reached out his hands to me and tears rolled down his cheeks. I held his hand and he said, "I have never felt peace like this before." Through story telling and sharing he was finding forgiveness and peace again, hope, and it helped me, too. Two weeks after he was released from the hospital I called him to ask how he was doing. He said, "My health is improving, I sleep better, the best thing that has happened is that I have become a happy grandpa; I wanted to make my grandchildren happy but I wasn't able to because I wasn't happy. Now I can make my grandkids happy." Telling a story has the power to heal.

When it comes to end of life, sharing stories with each other that are happy memories helps everyone. Sometimes people feel guilty about things they have done or not done, or about the decisions that are being made about patient care now. We have family conferences for critically ill patients where we discuss what kind of medical care should be given or withdrawn, shall we continue or not, and the palliative care specialist is part of that family meeting. The point that is emphasized is that whatever the decisions that are made are ones that need to respect the patient's wishes. But then, you always have to think about how far do you honor their wishes? Five years down the road are you going to be okay with your decisions, that you did everything according to his or her wishes, or that you withdrew life support too early?

Having advanced directives in place, and having these discussions with your family is so important. It's not easy, it is seldom black and white, you need to talk and prepare. Part of that preparation is to take care of unfinished business before it's too late, invest in building and enhancing relationships over your lifetime, and do good for others while you can. These are the things that I want to tell people about death.

Elaine
Registered Nurse
Bachelor of Science
University Adjunct Faculty in Nursing
Healing Touch Certified Practitioner
Certified Eden Energy Medicine Practitioner
Reiki Master

Introduction

Elaine was referred for the interview by Ben, the hospital chaplain whose interview immediately precedes this one. The benefits that he sees with Healing Touch led him to refer other practitioners, one of whom was Elaine, who works in the ICU of the hospital where he works. He knew that she would have a great deal of information about the benefits of energy healing for seriously ill and injured patients, as well as those transitioning from life into death. That certainly proved to be the case.

Interview

I have been a nurse for forty years and have attended thousands of deaths. My mother will tell you that I always wanted to be a nurse, that that was the only thing I talked about, but my dad will say that when I graduated from high school he told me I couldn't just sit around the house, that I had to get out and do something, so I applied to nursing school. In addition to my nursing degrees I am a Reiki Master, I completed the certification program with Donna Eden, I use kinesiology and meridian work, and I am a Healing Touch Certified Practitioner. I am also an adjunct faculty member at the local university nursing program.

My first introduction to Healing Touch was in the mid to late 1990s when a class was being offered here at the hospital and a girlfriend and I decided to do it. It just made sense to me, the philosophy, the understanding of being energetic beings just resonates for me, it makes total sense.

At that time in my life I didn't see energy move so clearly, I could see things but I think that came with nursing experience and practice and acceptance that we do have energy fields. I think anybody can see or sense things but our mind often covers it up or denies it because it is uncomfortable. For me it wasn't uncomfortable, it just felt natural.

As part of our training and our desire and need to practice, my friend and I offered some kind of technique to every coworker, every friend, and every family member we had. Some people gave feedback and some didn't. Everybody felt it, everybody changed, and it was reassuring and disarming at the same time for some because they had the experience but they couldn't explain it and it made them uncomfortable. I was too new at it and couldn't do a good job of explaining it to them.

For many years I didn't bring energy healing openly to my work but I do now. I offer my patients energy work by first asking them if they've ever heard of complementary therapies and what they have tried. I find that a lot of people who are toward the end of their life have explored a lot of things, so I ask them if they have heard of or tried Healing Touch or Reiki or any of the energy modalities that are really helpful with relaxation and centering. Some of them have, and some of them haven't, so I just tell them that I'm a practitioner in that field and I would like to offer that if they would like it and if they think it would be helpful. If they say yes I will do some energy work with them, and if they say no I just say okay, and we move along to whatever else they need.

One of the women I did Healing Touch with was in the ICU; she asked her nurse to have me come. We went in toward the end of our shift and I was doing some work with her, it was probably about forty minutes in when her son stepped into the room. I hadn't talked to him so I just kept working, and it was very, very beautiful and very soft. I finished up and stepped out of the room and he followed me and thanked me. He said when he stepped in there he could feel the love and the beauty that was surrounding his mom, and he appreciated it so much and would never have thought to ask for anything like that.

Sometimes I teach family members how to do some of the techniques. In helping people to feel more useful, in a time when they feel so helpless, I give them a little instruction and a demonstration on how to do some comforting techniques, just touch and intention, holding the heart space, and sweeping above and away from the body very gently to take away the pain. Because of my other training I usually explain to them which meridians come off the ends of your fingers and why holding the heart space with the tips of your fingers connects your heart to their heart which is comforting, it's always comforting, never bad.

Most people are totally trusting what you're helping them with because they feel so helpless, and since I'm in the trauma ICU as the experienced professional they are open to the suggestion of energy work. Some family members don't do it for very long because it's new to them and they have a little stage fright, feel a little awkward. The deep connection that can be made with energy work can also feel very intense to a family member, and it may bring up emotions they aren't always prepared to have viewed in such a public arena.

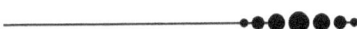

There are many conditions that energy healing helps alleviate such as pain, anxiety, agitation, and fear. I took care of a woman in the ICU who was screaming in pain and she had been given tons and tons of narcotics which weren't helping. I took a friend in with me and I said, "We need to do a session for her now, and we need to do a session every two hours for a total of three sessions." So we went in and did a session together, then I did two more sessions with her and after that she didn't need any more narcotics.

Most of the deaths that occur in this hospital occur in the ICU. We get everything that isn't cardiac; neurotrauma, surgeries, medical emergencies, accidents, and respiratory failures. I don't think that this hospital is different than any other hospital in that respect. Doing energy healing helps reduce anxiety significantly, and for that reason I think it brings them to a center, and when they enter that space people tell me that they float into a space where everything is good. It seems that it creates an opening into a space where they can relax into that centeredness of acceptance of the process. It does usually really help; it helps in the physical sense of struggle, the physical body seems to calm when you do energy work at the end of life, the respirations are more easy, the secretions become less, the person just appears more restful, more peaceful.

With energy healing you can slow a person's heart rate, can bring it down twenty or thirty points, bring the respiratory rate into a calm, even pattern, and bring their circulation back into their forebrain so they can have a rational thought instead of all those panicky, wild-eyed thoughts. Along with that comes a reduced need for medications, and one benefit of that is that the meds can make you crazy because as a side effect you may be experiencing hallucinations, things that are not you but are creating such fear and agitation.

There isn't a day that passes that we don't have a death in the ICU and how a person passes, energetically, is very easy for me to see now. It's hard to put words to, but there is a difference in the kind of death a person has depending on who their care person is, how afraid they are of death, and what beliefs they have about what happens after they die. If there is struggle it creates energetic chaos, and as a nurse and energy healing practitioner you have a really hard time getting hold of it and calming it. I think it comes from that space of fear. Our culture doesn't have an understanding of death, it's feared, we don't talk about it, we don't touch it, and we don't have it where we can see it. I've had people where I could calm that temporarily but I couldn't hold them there. There is some sort of emotional turmoil, maybe about relationships, maybe something spiritual going on. Energetically, the field seems chaotic, like the inability to find a space of peace. It might have to do with feeling that something is unfinished, incomplete.

A lot of times in the ICU when things are not going well, the doctors will say, "Go get Elaine, have her come and do that thing she does." They have no clue what it is, but it's "go get her, she needs to come and do that thing she does." Usually I'll just hold their crown, I'll just open that so they can go into that space where they're not anxious and I just stand in the space and hold their head and they're fine. It's crazy, but the docs seem to think it makes a difference.

When I am working with a person who is dying I hold their heart space because that connects for me who they are, and I always hold the second chakra. Usually their first chakra is gone, it's just still, as if disconnecting from the earth plane.[1] Sometimes the physical body will struggle on for a couple of hours as the energy body is disengaging because of the survival instinct, but I can feel their energy field getting bigger and bigger, I can feel it expanding, as the physical body is shutting down.

I will tell you a couple of stories that a person might call a good death, and I would say they were sacred experiences.

I was asked to see a young man who had brain cancer, had had it for a long time, had gone through all the processes, and he was in the end stages. He was in hospice and they had given him less than a week or so. His girlfriend was frantically looking for help, so his sister called me and said, "I know you do this, I don't know what it is." I think she called me just to appease the girlfriend.

So I went to their home and I set up my table in their bedroom. He was in a wheelchair and I got him up on the table. He had a brain stem glioblastoma so he could no longer walk, he had no control of his upper torso, and he was losing control of his secretions. He was gasping and choking on his secretions all the time, so lying flat, he thought, was going to be a challenge. But he was really cheerful and he was game, so I laid him on the table and he said, "Sometimes I have to clear my throat a lot," and I said, "Okay, I'll help you with that." So I started to work, and I just moved energy away from the body; the field was just really, really moist. At first he was clearing his throat and kind of having a hard time, but within ten or fifteen minutes it was all gone, it was good.

I never do just a part of a person, I always do their whole body, that's part of my training. I always open all of their meridians, so I opened him all up and I was just drawn to his head. So I was just pulling that energy away from his head, because he was having such headaches, such pain, just gently doing it, and it just got thicker and moister, and thicker and moister, and kind of rancid smelling. And then I thought that he blew a big breath on me, because my hair was long then, and my hair blew back. But when I looked down he was asleep, he was totally out of it.

And then the air began to move in the room. The curtains ruffled, I took a breath because I'm just a little bit disarmed and I'm thinking, "Okay, but I'm not sure you should die right now, I don't think they would like that very much." But I just gently kept working and it would stop, and then it would come back up again, like a burst of wind would just blow, and it would blow my hair back. I opened the window because it felt like it was getting so moist and thick in the room, like my hands were almost wet, and he was asleep, snoring just peacefully, beautiful, a beautiful young man, maybe about twenty-four years old.

So I just kept going, and when the energy field normalized and there was no longer that odd odor and it wasn't so thick, I just did the energy sweeps through the field, brushed him down and let him lay there for a few minutes, then I woke him up. He was sleepy, big pupils, starry-eyed. I got him off the table and laid him on the bed, and later his sister told me that he slept for about fourteen hours, which was something he hadn't done for weeks and weeks. He slept laying flat in bed, no more secretions, and when he woke up she said he was just so quiet. Before that he had been talking about going here, going there, somebody was going to fix it for him, but he was just so peaceful after he woke up. He visited with his family then went back to sleep and didn't struggle any more. He died a day or so later.

I asked a few people what they thought that was that blew my hair and ruffled the curtain, and one clergy person said he thought it was the angel of death. Our culture paints the angel of death as a dark, kind of icky figure, but there was nothing dark or icky about it, it was sweet, very sweet, but it was so unusual that I wondered what I was supposed to do, was I to stop the session? But the message I got was "Keep working, keep working, it will be fine. It will be just fine," said that little voice in my head, "you're exactly where you're supposed to be, just keep working."

Another time I went to a lady's home who had pancreatic cancer, an older lady, and I went there to give her pain relief because there was just no amount of narcotics that were helping her. I did a session with the patient and her angel was just so present. At the end I always just sit and talk with them as they're waking up, so we sat and talked for awhile. I didn't know anything about her, I had been called by a hospice nurse to come and do this for her. First we addressed her pain, no pain, she was perfectly comfortable. So I said, "Just lay here for awhile and talk with me." So I asked her, "Do you believe in angels?" and she said, "Well, I think so." I said, "I think I got to see yours, and she is incredibly beautiful. Have you ever had an experience with them?"

Then she started telling me about when she was a child when she had seen her angel. One time was when she had been on a piece of farm equipment and had fallen and her angel just sat with her until someone came. She also told me about how her angel would always come and talk to her at night. I think opening her chakras, where so much information is held about our lifetime, maybe that story telling eased her. I encouraged her to think about her angel now when she was falling asleep, or when she was uncomfortable, just think about your angel because she is right close to you. I said, "You know, if you saw her as a child, I bet if you asked you could see her again. She's beautiful." She smiled, she was just so sweet. Her poor sister, who had come to stay with her, didn't know what kind of look to put on her face. You get into that space when you're with somebody that you forget if there's anybody else in the room, but that was really sweet. She passed shortly after that.

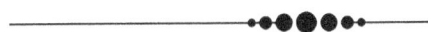

Near or at the time of death everyone has somebody come. Sometimes it's an auditory thing, almost like you hear conversations that you can't quite pick up going on in the room. Angelic presence isn't that winged, cloaked person, it's different for everyone. I guess that's what blows me away, it's different for everybody. Some people leave their body through their heart space and they just go up and you see like this light thing that goes off. Some people spiral, some people just kind of smolder out of their crown. I used to work with babies, and they go in kind of a little twinkle of a whoosh. I don't think babies are attached to being here yet, or something.

But there are lights, it's light, and it usually has some color but not always. I think that's an angelic presence. Sometimes it's an actual physical representation of a being at their bedside. I have often seen people sitting beside themselves, just kind of watching. A lot of times I will go in and talk to the patient when I know they are struggling, so I just go in and tell them what's going on. When people report going to the other side and coming back, or having conversations with someone in the room whom nobody else can see, I don't think they are hallucinating although family members often think they are. When we give too much drugs we cheat them out of their process, because I think it's an important process as an evolution of a being. Just like birthing is a process, dying is a process, and if we medicate them into not being present for it we're robbing them of that.

There is a big push now for assisted suicide, the Death With Dignity as the state of Oregon calls it. I've thought about it, but if people could understand that they could use things like Healing Touch and other processes that bring them into the center, that get rid of the pain, that eases the anxiety, then they might choose to go through the process of dying that way rather than skipping over it with assisted suicide.

The death of the young man with the glioblastoma and of the woman with pancreatic cancer, where they were able to go without pain and were physically and emotionally at ease, to me those deaths felt sacred. Even deaths when you're popped out of your body, like in an accident or something, when there's that sudden separation, I think there is a sacredness to that, but it must be a totally different experience.

The deaths that I would say where we've taken away the sacredness are deaths that occur in the ICU when we do what we call flogging, when the family doesn't want them to die, they want everything done, and we know that their body has failed and they can't survive, yet we will go on for weeks until it's just a mess, and in that suffering I think we lose the sacredness. I think the family suffers because their pain goes on and on, and the patients suffer, probably the patient suffers the least because they may detach and go somewhere else for awhile, kind of go back and forth. I think that's probably what they do, but the family definitely suffers, not knowingly making themselves suffer, but they do suffer and there's no sacredness in that. That's the worst part of my job, when I know we are promoting suffering.

We had one patient whom we knew had very little time left to live and that nothing we could do would prevent his death, but his son insisted that we continue with every procedure available even though they were useless and an assault on the elderly man's body. He had an advanced directive, the POLST form, and his wife kept insisting that this is not what her husband would want, that if he woke up he was going to be mad, but somehow the son's voice became the dominant one and, from my point of view, the doctors caved to the loudest voice.

The patient died eighteen days later, still in ICU, to the tune of $40,000.00 a day. It's a systems error; it's hard on the doctors, the nurses, the patient, and the family. In our culture we just can't seem to get a grasp on compassion being more important than technology, a compassionate death rather than a prolonged death.

In the field of medicine it seems that we have adopted the philosophy of whatever the family wants. I think we make an excuse not to step up as professionals in those situations. I think that we need to realize as professionals that they don't hold the knowledge card, we do. You don't have to be harsh with it, but there has to be those conversations. I don't know if it's just from exhaustion, or it's just emotionally too much, or it's our own stories that block us with being able to do that. I've sat with many parents when I worked with babies that were born so prematurely that their eyes were still fused and they had no skin yet, and I would say, "Oh, honey, I'm so sorry, but this is the situation and no matter what we do it is not going to be okay, so let's talk and decide what to do."

These can be agonizing conversations and we avoid them, I see physicians avoid them all the time. They'll come out and they'll say, "Well, they want just to keep going, but she's going to die." So why don't you sit down and explain that, then, in a way that they can understand? We don't have conversations in our culture that help us accept that the physical body eventually wears out, and with technology we seem to feel that we can avoid death, so when the family wants to keep pressing forward we may be able to do it but is it the right thing to do? As professionals it falls on us to help families through this, but we have to do it in ways that the family will understand. I see that the professional language, the medical terminology, can create real problems; it's like we're talking two different languages.

For example, when the family is asked, "What do you want?" the family will say, "We want her to survive, can she survive?" And the doctor will go, "Oh, yeah, she can survive." Well, what they are seeing is her sitting at the Thanksgiving table next year eating turkey: what the doctor is seeing is her living in a nursing home, drooling on herself. So the word "survivor" - we are not talking the same language. We may be talking about what they want, but we are not talking about the suffering that may well happen for the patient and the family for many years to come, taking someone home or being put in a nursing home who will never awaken again. We skirt around those issues because we have the technology to make it go on forever until everything truly does just totally collapse. And it's horribly expensive, financially expensive, and I think it's horribly emotionally expensive for the staff and for the families, and for the person who is trying to pass. If we knew we were going to work our whole lives so anything we were going to leave to our children would be eaten by our medical bills, would we choose that? No, most people wouldn't, but nobody wants to talk about that.

I've gotten really careful about how I talk to people because I think we're doing a disservice when we don't share the same meaning of a word or condition. A family member may come in and ask, "How are they doing?," and the response from the medical professional may be, "Oh, they're doing alright." What does that mean? Does that mean they can take the breathing tube out, that they are on their way to recovery, being able to breathe on their own, eat on their own, and come home before long? No, it probably doesn't mean that at all, so I have a responsibility to explain what the probabilities are in terms that the family can understand.

We need to be more open in our conversations about death, because not talking about it is not going to make it go away, it never has. We need to have conversations, because having those conversations will sweeten the experience, openly and without fear. I guess religion muddies that water a little bit sometimes because of some of the beliefs, but if we could come together as communities to talk about what end-of-life experiences look like, and how you want yours to be, it would be helpful. Do you want it to be in an ICU all wired up, do you want me to break all your ribs in an attempt to resuscitate you, do you want to be kept on machines until your urine looks like syrup, what do you want? Do you want to spend your whole life working so the hospital gets all your resources or do you want your children to have them? If you die unexpectedly at home, do you want the paramedics called whose mandate is to try to bring you back from the dead and then kept alive by machines in the ICU? Those are hard conversations to have because they sound so harsh in making those kinds of comparisons, but that's the truth. So we just need to talk about it, share, read the books by people who have crossed back and forth.

When I learned energy healing it changed how I looked at things and how I experienced them. I think that everybody holds the ability to help heal another, to bring relief and compassion to another, we just don't realize it. If people understood the importance of their energy body, how disease works, how powerful our minds are, how powerful the stories are that we tell ourselves, much of the disease that we experience wouldn't happen and we would experience less emotional distress as well. We're supposed to have experiences, it's always going to happen, but they could be more of an experience and a learning than a stress. We make things distressful when we don't have to. The energy healing, the Healing Touch, realizing that we're all so connected, that we're really powerful beings, it just doesn't have to be as hard as it is. I think what would make the biggest difference is that the energy healing shouldn't be the last resort,[2] and that's kind of where it's at now.

---

1. Chakras. Chakra is an ancient Sanskrit word meaning "wheel of light." It is believed that chakras act as localized energy distribution centers as well as centers in which one's life experiences are stored. There are seven major chakras located vertically along the spine. The first chakra is said to connect

us to the earth and some energy practitioners sense that this connection is broken as the death process proceeds, gradually shutting down each chakra as the physical system shuts down. The heart chakra is located in the middle of the chest and carries the energy of love.

2. All Healing Touch practitioners would agree with Elaine: energy healing should not be the last resort. A few hospitals and clinics offer Healing Touch by paid staff, but this is rare and it remains as a service largely provided by volunteers. Volunteers are not available as needed, they get burned out, they move; in other words there is no viable way yet established for patients to receive the care from which they could benefit. This leaves desperate patients, who have come to the end of what established medicine has been able to offer them, to reach out for something that will provide hope, help, and relief. Many of the complementary and alternative methods are offered while in hospice care, but why not before?

Mary Kay
Bachelors of Health Science in Physical Therapy
Guild Certified Feldenkrais Practitioner
Pilates Certified
Certified Healing Touch Practitioner and Instructor

Introduction

One hospital that has an integrative program that includes Healing Touch is the St. Luke's Medical Center, Wind River, in Ketchum, Idaho, where I interviewed Mary Kay. She started working at Wind River in 2002, managing the rehabilitation department. In 2009 when they were talking about starting an integrative therapies program she left that job to take the integrative therapies position.

Interview

The hospital had done a feasibility study and were looking for someone to run the integrative therapies program, and since it had been an interest and a passion of mine for so long it was a great fit for me.

At that time one of the doctors at the hospital was very into integrative medicine, and he and the woman who is the manager of a center for community health were funded to do the feasibility study. They looked at programs around the country and made recommendations on what modalities they thought would be best to start with: Healing Touch was one of the things they recommended.

It's a little surprising that Healing Touch was chosen as I would have thought that something better known like massage therapy would have been the initial offering, but in some ways massage is a lot more invasive than Healing Touch. There are a lot of people who don't want to be touched, or to have their bodies exposed, and those are not issues in receiving Healing Touch. I didn't know much about Healing Touch then except that it was an energy modality, but I had done some work with Donna Eden and loved it, so I was excited to get back into it.

At first it was a full-time position with a lot of the funding from the people in our community through our foundation. The first three years of the integrative therapy program was totally funded by the foundation and then that money ran out and it became operationalized under the hospital budget. As of now (2015), I have three main positions with St. Luke's: sixteen hours per week as the Healing Touch coordinator, about twelve hours per week doing physical therapy in the rehab department, and ten hours a week as co-chair on a Systems Integrative Therapies Steering Committee for all the hospitals and clinics in the St. Luke's system, trying to get integrative projects started and standardized across that system. These hours vary somewhat, of course, depending upon the need.

The timing for this to be happening now seems good. Nursing leadership is very supportive of integrative options as long as they are evidence based. Money to support the integrative programs don't necessarily have to come from the outside if you can find that you're saving a hospital money, if we get people out of the hospital sooner and decreasing costs. We started collecting data in 2009, and over that time the surveys show that patients received an average of a 50% reduction in pain and a 70% reduction in anxiety. We wanted to know how long those effects lasted and what we found is that they lasted anywhere from five minutes to a complete and permanent remission of pain. Five minutes does not sound like a lot, but patients were happy to have even that amount of relief. The caring and comfort care that they receive rather than just being poked and prodded, people truly taking their best interest and comfort in mind, I think that goes a long way.

Another big thing in medicine has become the patient satisfaction scores, (Hospital Consumer Assessment of Providers and Systems, HCAHPS for short) with the reimbursement from Medicare tied to these scores. So if you can show that you are affecting the score by using Healing Touch or other complementary modalities this saves the hospital money. Another way that could show cost savings is to do research to see if patients who receive Healing Touch and/or other modalities experience accelerated healing, decreases in medication use and costs, and earlier discharge with fewer readmissions.

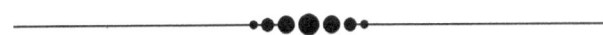

One of the amazing benefits to the hospital, the patients, and to the community is the number of people who have been trained in Healing Touch, with some going on for full certification. We are a small community, only about 20,000 in our valley, but we've had maybe ten Level I classes. These people end up treating their family and friends, and one of the spiritual centers has a weekly clinic where people can receive sessions for a donation. The classes, the sessions, and the sharing among practitioners and others who give and receive has brought people closer. I find it pretty amazing what it has done for our community. Anybody that I mention it to these days is familiar with it to some extent, either because they know somebody who does it, has taken a class, or has received a treatment. It's reminiscent of one of Janet Mentgen's stated missions, that somebody in every household knows how to do Healing Touch. We also offer free treatments for people in the medical community so they can experience the benefits first hand, and so they know what their patients are talking about when they say they are receiving Healing Touch.

One of our patients was here for palliative care and her whole family was coming from around the country to be with her. Her room was toward the end of one of the hallways and the family members were always holding vigil there, meeting outside the room and being with their loved ones. We have volunteers who come in six days a week to offer Healing Touch, and toward the end she may not even have known we were there as she was not responsive, but we did sessions anyway. We also offered it to her family members who were benefitting just as much as the patient if not more so. It was very grounding for the family and they appreciated that. Being there for everyone was a beautiful part of the process; it felt like we were able to nurture them and the patient through the transition.

Another woman and her family that were helped with the energy healing was someone I had known several years before when I took a class from her and now she was coming in for chemo infusion. This is another place that when people are just sitting in the chair or reclining, receiving their chemo infusion, I can do Healing Touch with them. This woman was having a lot of nausea and it was really beneficial for decreasing her nausea. I know that's a real common thing to use Healing Touch on, it's just not something that I had worked on a lot, I've worked more on pain and anxiety. So it was interesting to see how much the nausea was relieved by the Healing Touch. We have also begun to use aromatherapy tabs which are little packets of essential oils that are put on the patient's hospital gown. These are used for nausea and stress and anxiety reduction.

As her course of treatment continued she was in the hospital a few different times so I would see her there. On two occasions I also saw her husband, and he was a really interesting man. Both of them had taken workshops with Brugh Joy and he had great stories to tell about him. He was feeling very helpless about his wife's cancer and imminent passing, was having a harder time with it than she was, I think, so it was wonderful to see that doing the Healing Touch and letting him talk about his experiences, kind of recalling some of the things he had learned from Brugh Joy, was helpful for him in processing what he was going through.

She was amazing, she really wanted to show her children, her grown sons, how dignified death could be, and how graceful passing could be, so I think the energy healing played a role in that as well. And for all of them, just having people focus on their wellbeing and care, and the attention and the grounding in that time when things can feel so ungrounded, it was very helpful for all of them. In my opinion a peaceful death is one with no pain and little anxiety because the person has accepted that the end is near and they are ready to go. Patients and family members say that energy healing helps provide a peaceful death because pain and anxiety is decreased and relaxation and comfort is increased.

Even though I don't work with dying patients on a regular basis, I have gone to several palliative care conferences and at one of them I learned about the work of Stephen Jenkinson. The movie "Griefwalker"[1] was filmed over a twelve-year period about his work as a palliative care counselor. One of his main messages is that if we live with the knowledge that we will die and don't deny that fact, it allows for a richer life and more peaceful death.

Learning and practicing Healing Touch has made a huge difference in my life. It has taught me how to be present with people and allowed a means to do so. Being present has become kind of a buzz word, it's easy to say, but to truly be present is not always easy to do. I feel that it cuts through so many of the layers that are on the surface and allows you to truly connect with someone. Just the beauty of that is amazing.

There seems to be a dichotomy in the world today in that we are both more and less present with people. Technology definitely plays a role in that, both connecting us and keeping us distant. It can be hard and intimidating to truly show up for someone, to meet people in the world, to deal with social anxiety, but Healing Touch gives you a framework to be able to do that. It helps get down to the essential core, it doesn't have to be about talking, and that's even more beautiful because it cuts through all the layers of stuff that talking can obscure. It can be a truly spiritual experience.

In our training we are taught how important self-care is, so I meditate, exercise, walk in nature, do yoga, get massages, do self-Healing Touch treatments, get treatments from others, and travel. It has given me a greater awareness of myself, my own spirituality, and my own ability to listen to intuition and guidance from outside myself and within myself, and it all feels incredibly transformative. Watching this whole community of people here who have taken the classes together, who feel like it has changed their own lives so much, and to be a part of a community like that, it just kind of reverberates among the people and in the broader community, not just in myself.

When I think about what Healing Touch has done for our patients and their families, for people who have taken the classes and use it professionally or just on friends and family, and how much it has impacted me personally and professionally, I just have to say that it is an incredible gift.

---

1. Produced by the National Film Board of Canada in 2008, directed by Tim Wilson.

Jane
Registered Nurse
Certified Healing Touch Practitioner

Introduction

There are certain themes that have emerged from the interviews I have done and the discussions I have had, and one of those themes is the experience of Healing Touch being a gift to the practitioner and the recipients as Mary Kay described. Another theme is the burnout that nurses experience with the high tech nature of the profession now, which makes many of them feel that their purpose in becoming a nurse in order to connect and heal is not being met. It was not unusual for nurses to tell me that if they had not found Healing Touch and were not able to incorporate it into their nursing they would have quit the profession. Jane's story illustrates these points when she talks about the best and worst parts of her job. She brings a very strong religious and spiritual orientation to her story and to her work.

Interview

I have worked various positions in the hospital, but I work only in oncology now. We had a patient here from Hawaii who came for a bone marrow transplant and I was his nurse for several days. I did Healing Touch and he told almost everybody that his recovery was faster because of it, much faster than expected. That made me really, really happy.

I receive many comments and thank you notes from my patients. They say things like, "You are truly anointed by God for healing touch, that wonderful blessing and gift you have for healing." From another patient, "I had low platelets but after the Healing Touch they jumped from 26 to 51; amazing!" I also get comments from students who are with me such as, "Thank you for taking such good care of the patients," and from another, "Your kindness toward the patients is just amazing and you are really good at your profession. I am so grateful for being able to spend six shifts with you, to witness your organization and the Healing Touch."

Even before learning energy healing patients would say to me, "Your hands are different, your touch is different." I would ask them how. I spent some time in prayer and I asked God, "What is this? They are always talking about my touch. You need to show me what it is."

The doors kind of opened at the hospital when I heard about the Healing Touch classes being offered there; I was immediately interested and signed up for them. I loved it and wanted to do it professionally, so I decided to do all of the course work and the internship to become certified.

Before learning Healing Touch I would pray with and for people. I had a prayer partner and we always prayed for people. I sometimes called her to come to the hospital if I had a difficult patient who couldn't sleep or in some other way was suffering. She would come to the hospital and we would pray over the patient. I have seen some great results, but touching is really something different, you are exchanging energy.

I am in a prayer ministry now. That all takes a lot of energy and time, so before I go to pray with somebody I always need to spend time with God to recharge. You never know what kind of problem you are gong to face; that's why I always need His guidance and direction.

People have different belief systems around healing, but the way that I see it is that healing was Jesus' ministry and now I am doing His job. I should be proud of that. In the beginning my husband was totally against my doing this work, claiming that there is no such thing as universal energy, but as I can convey it more in terms of quantum physics he is understanding it.

Because we are Catholic I asked several priests about that, too, and they said, "If you touch people and invite Jesus into that, then you don't need to fear about anything." If I am using another kind of energy than I cannot do it, they said. Now, when I touch people, I invite

God and I want my hands to be His hands. That is what I am praying for. Jesus always touched people, and if I receive Holy Communion I am carrying Jesus with me, so my hands are His hands. So now I don't need to fear anything about it: I am not using any other kind of energy, I am using His energy, then why should I be afraid of it?

I have a friend who is kind of angry with me, too, because she told me that I am using a different kind of energy. I said, "I'm not. I talked to three different priests, and they are very well educated priests, and they all said the same thing: if I am using it in God's name I don't need to be afraid. I am not using any other energy, I am using His energy."

I do some free healing sessions for friends, but at the hospital it is integrated into my nursing work and there is no pay for it specifically. Right now the hospital administration says there is no money to fund a position, but if there ever is that is what I will do full time. I really want to go around and do Healing Touch, that's my passion now.

I use it for pain management and anxiety, fatigue, nausea, and to improve circulation and energy levels. It brings people into a calm state, their vital signs improve, they recover faster, and they may make a spiritual connection. Pain medications will often linger in the body for a long time, which affects the thinking, and Healing Touch helps clear it so the person is able to think more clearly. One time I had a patient with hiccups and he was hiccupping for days. I said, "I'm going to do something for you today. You just relax and I'm going to put my hands on you." Instantaneously it stopped, instantaneously. He was so amazed. His wife was there and she said, "I want that, too."

I will often do an energy scan in the course of the other nursing interventions that I am using, checking for things such as difference in temperature, for example. If I touch them I will tell them, "I'm putting my hands on you, or I'm touching different parts of your body and you may feel relaxation or different sensations." I let them know what I'm doing and the reason that I'm doing it. They can feel it, and the people who are present in the room can feel it, too.

One of my patients was a young man, only twenty years old, who was dying of cancer. He was a no-code patient, comfort care only, and I was blessed to be with him and give him Healing Touch at the end of his life. When I went in to do my shift the parents were hovering over him, so agitated, all over the place. So I sat with them, spent a lot of time with them, and I said, "Why don't you go to sleep; if there is anything I will call you, I will wake you up. He will be okay, I'm watching him."

So I stayed with him, did Healing Touch, and it helped him go peacefully from this world. He didn't have any agitation, nothing, just departed from this world so peacefully. I had never seen anything like that, such a peaceful death for a young guy. Usually they are all over the place, anxious, agitated, but this was a beautiful death. His parents were very appreciative and even named me in the obituary, calling me a "Healing Angel." These kinds of memories come back to me and give me a lot of strength, they keep me going. If I didn't see results I would quit, but I see and hear positive results day after day. It works, I don't have any doubts.

The young man I spoke of had a spiritual connection and I think that helped, too. When a person doesn't have a spiritual connection and fears the afterlife, or has unfinished business, unhealed relationships, what I have seen is that these people have more difficult deaths, and other nurses talk about this, too. If you have unresolved issues and you are on the pathway to leaving this world, you really need to resolve those issues, at least that's my opinion. Otherwise there is a resistance to going and nothing that we can do for them seems to work very well, not the medications, the prayers, or the Healing Touch. These are difficult deaths and the energy in the room feels bad.

One of my patients, a man in his 50s, wanted to have life, more life, more life, he did not want to go. So he was constantly asking the doctors, "Do you have anything else for me?" Sometimes the doctors have to say they don't have anything else and this patient and others like him then are so fearful, you can see how their faces change, the panic attack, and the anxiety in their eyes.

So, yes, I have seen both difficult and peaceful deaths. There have been times when I have been with a patient at the time of their death when I've heard heavenly music, and I encouraged the family to sing for the person who is dying because I knew their death was imminent. I told them that their transition should be a joyful event, the angels are singing for them, so why don't you join them? So one or two times

I had that kind of experience, or the room smells different, jasmine or something like that. And sometimes I have been able to feel very good energy in the room. With a peaceful death they don't have any fear to go.

When I can do the prayers and the Healing Touch with patients that is the best part of my job, but if I can't take any time with them, that is the worst. I need to be with them and I need to talk with them and I need to touch them, that is the best nursing I can do for them. If I just pass the pills out and don't have any time for them, what kind of nursing is that? On the days when we are so busy that it is just jumping from room to room, giving medications, hanging antibiotics, I say to myself, "What is this? I don't even have time for my patients." It does not feel good to me. When I go to work I want them to be energized, I want to see them healing, that makes me happy. Otherwise, it's just a mechanical thing I'm doing and no heart connection. That is not nursing for me, and this is nursing, Healing Touch. I need to touch people, I need to be with them, I need to be part of their life; that's nursing for me.

Marty
Bachelor of Science in Nursing
Master of Science in Nursing
PhD in Adult Organizational Learning
Advanced Holistic Nurse - Board Certified
Associate Professor of Nursing
Certified Nurse Educator
Hospital Integrative Medicine Staff
Certified Healing Touch Practitioner

Introduction

When I was looking for Healing Touch practitioners to interview for the book I was thrilled to find Marty. With her credentials, years of work as a nurse and as an instructor, supervision of students doing hospital rotations, serving on dissertation committees, presenting workshops for nursing continuing education, her integration of Healing Touch into her work, and her Level 5 mentoring of nurses working toward their certification, I felt as if I had struck gold.

Marty was hugely helpful in suggesting people to interview for the book. I began to refer to her as the hub of a wheel with the spokes going out in all directions with the people that she suggested for interviews and the connections that she helped me make.

Jane, whose interview appears right before Marty's, is one of the nurses that she said I absolutely had to interview. Because of the accolades that Jane modestly mentioned in our interview, the reference in the young man's obituary to her being a "healing angel," it brought a public affirmation not only to her, but to every Healing Touch practitioner about the value of our work.

Since the interview Marty has retired from her university position so some of the statements about her work need to be read in the context of this change in her academic status.

Interview

Becoming a nurse seemed like a natural progression and good fit for me, from having a mom who is a nurse, being good at science, and interested in helping people. It's been a really rewarding profession for me. I worked in the critical care area for many years and was recognized for my expertise there, and for a number of years taught courses on critical care. I was asked to precept some students in the critical care area, and then I was asked to teach at the university. I was adjunct faculty there for awhile, went back to school to get my masters degree, and with that I moved into more full-time teaching, so I have been in a teaching position for over twenty-five years.

I was introduced to the concept of energy healing by a nurse colleague who was working with me in intensive care. One evening I took a report from her about a patient who had an abscess below his pancreas. He had been suffering from confusion and irritability and was in a lot of pain. He was in isolation, and I will never forget getting the report that he had been unable to sleep for a really long time, like for a day or so.

My colleague said, "I watched a video and I was going to do this energy work with him." She described how you center yourself, you go to that still point inside, and even though this was the first time I had ever heard about energy work I thought, "I know where that still point is." She described the process of centering, then focusing on the patient, then drawing your hands down over the patient a few inches above their body, and focusing on the areas of warmth or tingling or coolness, and then just smoothing that out with your hands. So I thought, "That sounds interesting," and decided to try it. I was really happy that I was in the isolation unit because you can pull the curtains and nobody can see what you are doing.

I assessed the patient and he was in a lot of pain; wasn't able to verbalize what was going on, very agitated and moving around. I got the morphine and gave that to him intravenously and then I thought, "I'll do this thing that she described." I did the centering and grounding as she described, then I did this process of Healing Touch where you run your hands through the energy field a few inches above the body, and found that there was a great deal of warmth over the area where the abscess was. After that I again spent some time running my hands a few inches above the body to smooth out the energy field. When I was done I quietly stepped out of the room and he slept for four hours. I thought, "What just happened here?"

It was really easy for her to describe it and for me to do it. After that I was in contact with a couple of other nurses who had heard of this Healing Touch, and there were courses in the area, so we went to the trainings. I went through two levels, then practiced off and on as I could, but people knew that I was able to do Healing Touch and asked me to help them out. Eventually I went through all the levels and received certification. I got connected with Mary Kay (see her interview) and she invited me to do a research project with some other nurses, so I was a mentor for that group.

When I started teaching holistic nursing I would teach aspects of Healing Touch within the course, I was known for that. I have been teaching that class for about fifteen years, so it's been going on for quite awhile. After taking Healing Touch classes I was then able to teach the very basics for the students to get an awareness of the process. These were not classes that would lead to certification, just basic information and rudimentary skills.

When I first started doing Healing Touch and teaching basics at school, I remember friends asking me to "Do that voodoo that you do," so there was a lot of skepticism. I was happy when there was more research being done to support it, and more and more nurses starting to recognize the impact of it, how it felt when I would work on them, and how their patients would respond. For instance, one semester we had a student who had a patient who was on the neurological floor, in so much pain, so I went in and just did a chakra connection and after that he rested comfortably. They were amazed, and the nurse turned to me and said, "I've got to learn that." So it just passes from one nurse to the next.

The research study that Mary Kay and I coordinated was on measuring the effects of Healing Touch on recovery on outpatient surgical patients, mostly on orthopedic patients. They were randomly assigned to receive standard nursing care or standard nursing care with Healing Touch added. It showed that the patients who received Healing Touch got a fairly significant reduction in their need for medication. Often after surgery patients will have trouble with bowel and bladder functions and we didn't include outcome measurements for these, but Healing Touch is relaxing, and often as patients relax their other functions improve. I have found reflexology to be really effective in stimulating bowel functions.

Since most of my work is teaching and mentoring, I have not been with very many patients during their death process. Occasionally there will be a patient that the students might have in end-of-life care and they ask me to be involved, but the most significant deaths for me weren't those of patients but of my father and father-in- law. Both my dad and father-in-law were in assisted living facilities and I went to their bedsides, which was really very important, an honored kind of place to be. Both these times were very significant moments in my life, or poignant I guess the word would be, to be able to offer this work. My dad was very agitated, and my father-in-law was also not resting well, so with both of them I was able to do the chakra spread. It was one of the things that was very helpful to them, to be able to relax, breathe easier, and allow the process to happen, to allow themselves to go.

I think when I first got comfortable with end of life was listening to Elizabeth Kubler-Ross. My mother was teaching at a community college in the LPN program, and at one point she had Kubler-Ross come in as one of her speakers. I was in an undergraduate college program in another town at the time but I went home specifically so that I could hear her. Listening to her talk about how people feel and what they need at end of life, how oftentimes they hold on and don't let go until something specific comes along to help with that transition, all of that was very interesting to me.

And then, my mother stayed so close to end-of-life care, and I feel as if her way of doing things was really an inspiration for me, as well; her comfort with people, her being able to sit with them at the end of their lives. So when I was with my dad and my father-in-law it was just sort of a natural way to be. I think I would probably have done more Healing Touch with both, I was able to do some with them, but I would probably have done more had I been more part of a group and if there had been more emphasis on it like there is now. I knew how to do it, and knew how healing just being present is, but the use of Healing Touch really came later for me. I feel as if that would be an excellent calling, to be like our friend Jane, being in the center at end of life and being able to be very impactful for someone during that time. But I have been able to use Healing Touch with people with very severe conditions and help them be more comfortable, both in my private practice and in the hospital.

Some of the agitation at the end of life, I can't ever be sure if it is physical, emotional, spiritual, or a combination of all three. I think my father felt that he was not in a good place spiritually, and I think that may have been some of his agitation, almost like it was painful for him to release, so he held on for quite a long time. When I watched him his face was really tense and tight. With Parkinson's, a lot of the time, it really affects the facial features, they're kind of flaccid or almost frozen, but he almost had a frown on his face so I was trying to work to relax him and talk to him about letting go, that it would be okay. Eventually he did let go, I actually think the last dose of morphine that the nurse rubbed into the mucous membrane on the inner cheek took him with little ability to do much more holding on.

As I've watched people at the end of their lives, whether family members or others, whether we're using Healing Touch or not, if they have already come to terms about what's going on, then there is this transition that comes over people of ease and peace. I feel as if my father had some fear. There was a great deal of resistance, his face had this painful look like he didn't really want to go, yet when it was time and he went there was a whole different look. Of course the spirit wasn't there, and then you get messages later on, after death, that he was okay. There were some things that had occurred during his life that I think he was concerned about and was hoping that we would be alright. I think he was almost asking for forgiveness, which was easy to do, because I forgave him a long time ago. So I would tell people to come to terms with their life and their death and not to be afraid.

When I've been in the room at the time of a death there is a shift, sort of a difference in lightness in the room, as if something had been let go. With my father-in-law it was really a nice feeling. He was a very spiritual man, his Catholicism was very strong, so he led a very good life. His death was different than my dad's, just really relaxed, you could just feel that he was leaving, almost like a draft of energy and then he was gone.

I had a nephew who was born with a hypoplastic left ventricle and he lived for about forty-eight hours. I was able to hold him for a couple of hours before he passed, but I was at home when he passed and the next day I woke up and I could just smell him, like he was coming by to say goodbye. Then when I talked to his mother, my sister-in-law later that day, she said she was walking through her kitchen and she said, "I could feel him, I could smell him." I told her I had had the same experience, it's as if he was saying goodbye.

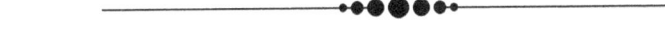

As a clinical instructor I was able to go in to see the patients with the students and show them how to make the patient comfortable with Healing Touch. In my private practice I've seen people with different stages of pain, and maybe an illness they're trying to work through, and it's just amazing. Well, you know how Healing Touch is, how it can help people be more comfortable with just the smallest things. It's difficult to explain, almost; you have to experience it to really understand it.

I was with someone the other day who had already gone through breast cancer treatment and during that time I was able to help her in a guided imagery group and at various other points in her recovery. At the last week of our guided imagery group she texted me that she wouldn't be able to come because she had gone to see her physician and had gotten a diagnosis of bladder cancer. So she had had surgery already where they attempted to remove as much of the tumor in the breast as they could, but then she was facing having surgery to have her bladder removed.

We did Healing Touch which was very relaxing for her, very peaceful, helping her focus. She wasn't in pain at the time but of course she was experiencing anxiety over what to expect for the bladder cancer. I talked to her for a little bit about the catheter that she would probably be using, that it's another way of elimination, we discussed what that might be like for her, and what kind of information she would be receiving from the doctor and nurses as she went along. It was a nice connection for her and she texted me to say thank you.

Two of the other clients that I worked with in my private practice, both cancer patients, benefited from the energy healing work as they were going through their regular treatment. The first client had breast cancer and I did a combination of massage and Healing Touch for her prior to her surgery and then again afterwards. She was able to choose where she would go for surgery and for chemotherapy and the other follow-up procedures that she needed. She did all of her follow-up religiously, she's very good about doing those kinds of things and now, over five years later, she's still going strong. The ability to have choices and control I feel is important.

The second client had ovarian cancer and I was able to do energy healing with her as well as some of the trauma work that we are taught in Healing Touch. Her story is one of a series of accidents that required medical treatment which led to her cancer diagnosis, and without the accidents she might not have been diagnosed early enough for a good recovery. It changed the course of her life and she is now doing healing and bodywork. Sometimes the events in our lives that we initially think are the worst things that could happen redirect our lives in ways we could not have imagined and it turns out to be quite wonderful.

I believe that the more people who experience the work, and the more who talk about it, the more it will become incorporated into mainstream medicine. Patients are going to ask for it because they are not all about medications, they don't want to take medications and deal with the side effects, and sometimes medications don't do the job. One of my students had a patient who had significant pain that was not being controlled and he was asking for more and more medication. This student and her nursing supervisor asked me to come in and do Healing Touch, so I went in and did a couple of the interventions for relaxation and pain reduction and he fell asleep during the treatment. They were all amazed at the results and later he asked me to teach his wife how to do it. He wasn't completely pain free, but it made a huge difference in how he was feeling and the fact that he got some sleep. So again, it is important to allow people to experience it, see the difference it makes, and share that information.

Working with hospitalized patients usually has constraints that are not there when I work with someone in my private practice. When I do a session I have music on, I have scented candles, sometimes I use lotion, I'll do guided imagery, talk them through a healthful way of being, see themselves, feel themselves, what would you feel around you, what would you hear, what would you see, what would you taste, guiding them in using all the senses. Being a completely healthy person, what would touch feel like, what would it smell like, I might also ask that. So the more senses that you use to visualize the outcome the more powerful it can be.

As far as how it has impacted me as a person and a professional since learning Healing Touch, it truly has been the core and the center of what I do. I feel like I want to reach out to everybody, help everyone, because I know how powerful it is, how touch can affect people, how the energies around us can affect people. Just talking about it doesn't really describe how the body, mind, and spirit has integrated, has just shifted to health and wellbeing. When I'm working with someone and the outcome that we want is pain reduction, for example, and I want them to be healed of their symptoms that they came to me for, and the outcome doesn't happen, I have to have a little talk with myself, I have to remind myself that this may be their path and not to get my ego involved in it. I remember hearing early on in our courses to get the ego out of it, and truly that is very important. When I can help people I feel like it fills up a lot of the qualities I have in my heart and mind, the heart center of where I come from wanting to help people, and knowing that I can with Healing Touch.

It has changed my life to be teaching Healing Touch and mentoring nurses who are working toward certification. The certification brings recognition of the ability to go through all five levels. Being able to teach the rudiments and bring the awareness to my students in the holistic nursing classes has been very important to me. I've spread the word to hundreds of students that way, many aspects of holistic nursing, so I feel I've really influenced a lot of people, that this is very meaningful in helping increase the awareness of these modalities. I have used Healing Touch on so many people; friends, family, clients, patients, it's just a gift where you are giving and receiving at the same time. It has changed my life.

Terry
Bachelor of Science in Nursing
Healing Touch Practitioner
Usui and Karuna Reiki Master and Teacher
Eden Energy Medicine Certified Practitioner

Introduction

Terry is a retired nurse after forty-four years, much of it as a critical care nurse. She is now in private practice as an energy healer using Healing Touch, Reiki, Donna Eden energy medicine, and Ortho-Bionomy. We see in some of her stories the challenges of working with the most seriously injured and critically ill patients, and both the benefits and the limitations of using energy healing in these cases. She also addresses the issue of communication between doctors, patients, and families.

Interview

I was first introduced to Healing Touch when I went back to school to get my Bachelor of Science in Nursing. There was a Therapeutic Touch class that was part of the nursing electives and I thought it would be an easy class, but it really opened my eyes to energy healing and I liked it, I'm glad I took it. Then I took the Healing Touch classes that were being offered in my area and began using it with my patients in the critical care unit.

I would use it a lot on people who were very confused, or people who were having a lot of pain and the meds just weren't controlling it. It seemed to help them relax somewhat, as long as I was standing there, but they couldn't hold the energy if I wasn't standing in the room with them. Even if I wasn't touching them but just standing there and projecting a healing presence they seemed to be much quieter, but then it didn't take much time at all for them to revert to their symptoms of confusion and pain.

For people who were very combative, it helped if I did something to hold their head and their heart, to do a connection between there, that seemed to be helpful and they would quiet down some. If they were given pain medication, the medication seemed to help them quicker if I did work on them. I found that head injuries were very difficult. A lot of times I would feel them pushing back, their energy pushing me away, if I was up around their head. If I was around their body that was okay, but if I got around their head at all it felt like they pushed out and you could feel the energy field sometimes just radiating. They were a little more difficult because it seemed like their energy was so disconnected, it was just chaotic around their head. They would settle some if I worked on their body, but it was a lot of work.

Sometimes it wasn't the patient who was agitated, it was the family. I remember one cancer patient with many of his family members in the room and they were at odds with each other, not so much about him dying but what he had done, it was all of this stuff that people tend to drag up when they are so agitated about something and they have no control. They sounded so very angry and I thought, "This is not going to help my patient at all." So I went to the door and I just stood there and filled the room with energy, that was my intention, to just fill the room with healing energy and just to let that permeate everyone and everything in the room. It only took about five minutes, they quieted down, and they were just sitting there talking, reminiscing about when they were kids on vacation, and so on. The conversation had changed so much. One of the doctors came up and asked, "What are you doing?" and I said, "Just filling up this room." He said, "Oh, you're doing that thing again," and walked off. He came back later and said, "It kind of worked, didn't it?" and I said, "It kind of did." But it was such a change in the atmosphere of the room, just filling it up. You don't have to work on just one person, you can do a lot with just intention and with moving that energy into that space.

When I would do energy work with patients, even if they were comatose or heavily sedated or in a chaotic, confused state because of a head injury, I would introduce myself and tell them what I was going to do. I would just say to them, "I have something that will help with your stress and with any anxiety that you have, and help you with your pain. If you don't want this you can let me know." I have had people push me back, or it would be like working on the desk, there just wasn't any movement, and I would say, "Okay, I understand, I'll offer it to you again later."

I had a very big "aha" moment early in my Healing Touch career. I had a nurse come to me in the middle of the night, "The patient is having trouble with his inner cranial pressure, can you come down and do that thing that you do so I don't have to call the neurosurgeon?" I said, "You're still going to have to call the doctor, but yes, I will come down there."

I went down and I didn't do what I usually did, I didn't say to him, "I'm Terry, a nurse here, and I'm going to offer you a Healing Touch treatment and it will help you feel better." Without gaining or sensing his permission I just went in and started working because my intention was to help the nurse and to help the patient, but as soon as I got close to him and positioned my hands to do the treatment it was like hitting a brick wall. I thought, "Oh, it's not working!" But then I thought, "Oh my gosh, I am so sorry." I hadn't explained what I was doing, so I explained it to him, and as soon as I explained and introduced myself and said what I was going to do then it was different, it was just night and day difference. I knew he wasn't intentionally blocking the energy because he was comatose, his intracranial pressure was high, he was on the ventilator, so I knew it wasn't his conscious self that was blocking, it was his Higher Self saying, "No, that's not the way to do it." His intracranial pressure came down and he did better the rest of the night.

In my hospital the nurses who have experience with Healing Touch feel comfortable asking for it for patients, but the doctors have been told that they cannot offer alternative, complementary, or integrative therapies. If a patient brings it up then they can make a referral, but they cannot initiate the conversation. The chaplains can bring it up, but not all chaplains believe that humans have an energy field that can be affected by energy healing modalities.

But what I want to say is that people heal themselves, that the body takes the energy of the treatments and uses it to heal themselves. We are all composed of energy, the things that hold us together is energy, and when we go down to our atoms they are held together with energy, our whole body is made up of that energetic process. Our heart, our brain, everything has an energy to it, it's electrical and it moves, and if it doesn't move like it's supposed to then we have problems. Physicians use transcutaneous electrical nerve stimulators (TENS) units, devices that are energy modalities used to treat pain, magnets are used for non-unions when a bone won't heal, so I feel that energy therapies, no matter what they are, can be an integrative and complementary piece of any kind of treatment for a patient.

If I had a broken leg, yes, I would definitely have somebody fix that, put it back together, and then I would have somebody do energy work so that healing would happen quicker. It seems that once doctors saw the effectiveness of the work they would want to integrate it into their treatments. The cardiologists who have one of the nurses give Healing Touch to their patients have great success: healings are better, their grafts work out better, their patients are happier and have an easier time of it than the ones who don't receive the energy healing work.

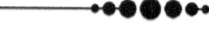

Because of the units I have worked in I have seen many deaths, some that I would say were easy, maybe you could call them good deaths, and some that were bad because they were hard and there was such a struggle.

We had an experience in the unit, it was a man who had spent the day fighting something. He was dying, you could see it and all his vital signs were pointing to it. As the shifts were changing, the day shift reported that "He's been fighting all day, there's something in there he's fighting with. He's talking to things that aren't there, he's talking to people who aren't there, and he's just really having a difficult time." He was scared, you could see it on his face, and when you walked into the room you just felt like there was something bad in the room, it just wasn't a good feeling. People would say, "I'm not going in there by myself, I want someone to come with me," it was that obvious, people who would never say that. I even had a doctor say, "Come with me, there's something weird in here."

The patient was talking to someone that we couldn't see, begging, pleading, arguing; it was just very sad to see this person have such a difficult time. When he died, which was in the late evening, the crucifix in the room turned upside down and fell off the wall. So we really didn't know if he was taken, if the bad guys got him, if the good guys got him, if he ever made that escape transition or what happened. When the priest came up the next morning to see another patient we said, "We know that you can't do an exorcism or anything like that, but if you would just go in and bless the room it would be helpful, please." Even the people who came to clean up the room from housekeeping were not comfortable in there. They came out a couple of times and asked, "What happened to the man who was in here?" I asked them why they were asking, and they said, "I don't know, it's just wrong."

Sometimes medications can create hallucinations, but this was different, it wasn't that. So when I think of a hard death, or a bad death I think about his, it was very difficult. He was fighting the whole day, it was something to see, something you don't want to see. Sometimes I think of a bad death as one that happens very quickly, but on the other hand it might be a good death for it to happen that way because the person doesn't have to suffer like this man did, or in other cases be kept alive through heroics because of families not willing to let go.

In science we don't talk about things like energy attachments, but I remember two cases where it seemed that the energy I was working with wasn't the patient's. We had a young man brought in from a rollover car accident, the car had rolled over a couple of times and he had been thrown out. I remember him so well for a couple of reasons. The first is because he had been injured so badly with head and chest injuries; there was severe swelling in the brain and the outcome didn't look good.

A year and a half or so prior to the accident there had been a crisis in his life and it was just like all of a sudden all of the bad juju that he could dream up, he did. He drank, did drugs, drove too fast; he worried his mom to death. We were waiting on her to come, and when

I put my hands on his feet with the intention of raising the energy up through his body to stop the bleeding from his head and help him settle I thought, "There's something not right about you." Just that brief contact and it was like his energy crawled up my arm and it took me over two hours to get it off. I did do some off the body work in his energy field, but his energy was so chaotic my arms felt like things were running up and down them, just clawing almost. I couldn't make it quit, I couldn't get it off. He was so afraid, and finally when I got him settled and I put my hand on his heart I said, "It's going to be okay, your mom's on the way, she'll be here soon and you're going to be fine. Whatever it was you're running from you're safe now," and he died. He just kind of quit, his heart hadn't stopped yet, but he just kind of quit, his breathing stopped, everything just stopped.

The other case was a man who was a dare devil and he was jumping over a number of semis with his motorcycle. He hit the last one, and his energy field was like the young man's, it just acted like it wanted to grab everything. His sister said he would like to have energy work, and when I touched him to tell him what I was going to do it was like something just crawled up all over me. I said "Stop it, go away!" It took me a while to get that off of me, whatever that was, but it definitely felt really nasty, assaultive almost. I don't think it was actually him, I think it was something else.

One of the best parts of my job is when I have time to be with the family of a patient, spend time in the room with them or just be available. Sometimes a person does not go through the agonal breathing pattern[1] that precedes death, maybe they've been taken off the vent and they've just stopped altogether. It can be very difficult for the families to all of a sudden feel like they're finally gone, and they might be questioning whether or not they did everything they could. I have a conversation with them, tell them how well they did, how they were there for the person, how much they must care for this person to witness their final moments because it's very important, and they did all they could do. It's important that they hear somebody say that to them, somebody who's been around and understands this part of the death process. Having people share more about who this person was, what he or she did, sometimes just having them share memories is very helpful to the family and it's helpful to us as nursing staff, too, because it helps us understand more about how the family is feeling and how we may be able to support them.

One of the worst parts of my job is when a patient is dying, is ready to die, and a family member simply can't let go. Sometimes family members have been estranged and the person with the decision-making power hasn't seen the dying person for years, yet they have to make the final decisions. It is usually a shock for them to see the condition their family member is in, and with so much unfinished business there are emotions that are swirling around making it hard to come to a rational decision. I try to help them by asking what they think the patient would want, not what they want, but they may not know. Don't wait until the last minute: if there is somebody you haven't seen in years and you will be involved in some manner at the end of their life, give them a call, have a conversation. The situations where nobody knows what the dying person wants, where there is so much unfinished business, is hard on everybody.

As professionals I think we have a responsibility to ask some of the difficult questions and help the decision makers see what the patient may or may not have wanted at end of life. We can tell them the probable outcomes of procedures or of just providing comfort care, and ask what the patient may have already shared with family and friends. I may ask, "Have you ever had a conversation with them about what they wanted; what did they tell you?" They may have made statements such as, "I never want to live like that," or "I never want to be like this." Would your loved one want to live if they were in a vegetative state, kept alive by machines? Knowing how to ask the right questions is very important. So many times the doctors will ask the question "What do you want?" but that's not the right question. The right question is what the patient wanted, and if the family knows that they can honor those wishes, and when they look back they can have comfort in knowing that they did what their loved one wanted.

We had one patient whose family had moved to the United States from another country. The wife was the patient, and the doctor kept asking the husband, "What do you want to do?" Of course he wanted his wife to live, but finally one of the nurses asked him, "In your country, who makes this decision?" He said, "Where I am from the doctor comes and tells you, ' your wife is going to die,' they know these things, I don't, I would never want her to die, but when the doctors here ask, 'do you want to stop this?' – 'no, I want her to live.' But if the doctor came to me and said, 'she is so sick we cannot make her well, and she is going to die,' then I would understand, but that's not the question that they would ask me."

Lack of information, guilt, unfinished business, belief systems, all of these can play a role in what decisions are made and how they are made. I knew a doctor who did everything for his patients because he could not let them die, let alone die a peaceful death. I found out after taking care of some of his patients that he believed that once a person dies that's it, there is no afterlife and you are gone from the universe as if you never existed, so he had to keep his patients alive at any cost. So he just kept pushing to the edge and then pushed some more.

For a lot of people it's a relief, they're done and they know it. They may be more comfortable than the people standing around the bed. Death isn't the worst thing, sometimes prolonging life is. For whatever reasons, people think that the death process is horrible. We tend to drug our people, so they are kind of in oblivion when they take their last breath. I know there's fear involved, and I know people get anxious, but I also know that for a lot of people when they die they open their eyes wide, like "I want to see this! Oh, I'm going someplace!" they have that look to them. Why would I want to give them medication to obliterate that possibility of them being able to see whatever it is that they're seeing? I think that we think too often that it's more painful if they're doing these things, and we tend to want to make it easier on the family who's sitting there, so we take that all away. I think that we do that a little bit too freely and we're encouraged to, I think that might be a problem, but it's easy to give a shot and then just walk out of the room. Sometimes that's all you can do if you're busy with other patients and it makes the family feel like you've fixed it.

If somebody is in an unusual breathing pattern, the tendency will be for the family to ask for something, or the nursing staff will give the patient something so that he or she doesn't have to work so hard, try so hard to breathe. People need to be educated, to know that this is how people often look when they die, this is what happens, this is the physical part of it, it's not that they just close their eyes and they're gone. Sometimes we need to talk about that, but people find it very gruesome, or morbid, but I think there is a certain amount of information that needs to be given about the dying process.

Sometimes Healing Touch can ease that process, can make the breathing a little easier, and we can have the family join in by telling them where they can put their hands and how everyone can join their energies to relax the patient, to take the fearfulness out of the process for patient and family, to take away the anxiety so the patient is more at ease. I think that would be better than using too much medication.

It's not unusual for the family to have held vigil for hours if not days, and the one time everybody is gone from the room the patient dies. People feel guilty that their loved one died alone, but for some that seems to be exactly how they wanted it. For others, they don't want to be alone. I had a patient who was severely injured and before I went off duty that day I said, "I'll be back at 3:00 tomorrow, you just hang in there." The next day I went in at 3:00 and said, "Hi, it's Terry, I told you I'd be back," and he died. I thought to myself, "You didn't have to wait," but that's what he wanted, somebody to be witness to his death. I think that being a witness at that time, and being present, *really* being present for them, not just showing up, is huge.

In addition to the ways Healing Touch helps my patients and their families, becoming a Healing Touch practitioner has made me more patient, both professionally and personally, and given me a broader perspective on life and death. I think I am more at peace with the idea of death and dying, how things progress, and not knowing the answers to the journey we call life is okay, more trust in the process. I'm more optimistic, more tolerant, nothing is cut and dried, nothing is the end of the world. I can talk to my grandchildren in a different way, helping them see events from different angles, and always working on more compassionate caring and conversations in all of my interactions.

---

1. Agonal breathing is an abnormal pattern of breathing characterized by gasping, labored breathing. The person makes sounds and may twitch and jerk.

Lilli
Bachelor of Science in Music Education
Massage Therapist
Reiki Practitioner
Ortho-Bionic Practitioner
Healing Touch Practitioner

Introduction

Lilli is an example of how combining energy healing methods with other training and skills enables one to create a synergistic practice pleasing to both clients and practitioners. She is also a wonderful testimony to how doing what you love has no age limit, and in fact probably helps a great deal at keeping a person young in body, mind, and spirit. At the time of our interview she was within one month of celebrating her 85th birthday. Her path to energy healing wasn't a straight one, it seldom is, which she shares in her story. She does not work in end-of-life care but her stories illustrate how energy work can be used in physical, emotional, and spiritual healing.

Interview

How did I get into Healing Touch? Well, here's the story.

I had started massage, and I had a friend who said, "You need to take this class." I had heard about Healing Touch in my massage work and I thought it was too far out, but since Marty (see Marty's story) was bringing this class I would take it for her sake, to support her. I took the class but I didn't use it because I thought my clients would think I was a little bit crazy. And then one day, I had a gal that came in every week, and she was yakking away and I thought this is not like her, so I said to myself, "I'll just do a chakra connection." When I moved my hand from the knee to the hip she said, "I don't know what you're doing, but it's very relaxing." I thought, "Well, you don't have to tell people what you're doing." So I started using it, every massage that I did, I made sure they were relaxed by using Healing Touch as part of the session.

Then I took the second and the third class fairly close together, and from that point on I was sold on it. I went to Hawaii for my Level 5 instruction which begins the one-year mentored internship leading to certification, and there I met Janet Mentgen, founder of the Healing Touch Program™. We chose partners for the week and were also assigned to a certified practitioner who would go into Queen's Medical Center every day. I was assigned to a man and his wife, he was an instructor, and he told me that he took a Level I Healing Touch class to prove that his wife was wrong about energy work, that there was nothing to it, but after about half an hour he started to see auras and quickly changed his mind.

The first person that we saw in the hospital was a woman whom he had been doing sessions with for a few days and she said, "I'm so glad you're here; it's going to be an hour before I can take any pain medication." She had had her foot amputated above the ankle. He started working on her, she relaxed and went to sleep and remained sound asleep for a good 45 minutes, I would guess. I thought, "Oh, my word." I had never worked on anybody like that. He saw four or five other people that day, but I don't remember any of the rest of them, she's the one that stuck in my mind. That was a real eye-opener as far as offering energy healing in hospitals was concerned. From there I started using it all the time, of course, often combining it with other modalities including Reiki and Ortho-Bionomy.

Ortho-Bionomy is a method of gently moving parts of the body to relieve pain and to remind it that it can move back into balance and heal. Ortho means bone, bionomy means balance. We don't believe in causing pain, so if people are in pain we stop because we are doing something wrong. It's perfect for older people who are in pain so many times, so along with the Healing Touch it's just fabulous, it's great.

Anyway, the first story I'll share is about this gal who came for massage every week, it was a Thursday afternoon, and during the massage she told me that she and her husband were flying to Florida the next day and she had to go home and pack for herself, her husband, and her sons. So I said I had just learned a Healing Touch technique which would help her stay focused, everything she needed to get done would get done easily, and then she could just sit back and relax. That's exactly what happened she reported later, but when I started the work what I felt was very odd.

This technique I used is done by holding points on the head and face, and during the first position my hands got extremely hot and there was a buzzing, I can't explain it any better than that, so I just held the position until the heat dissipated. It was the same with every position: I would wait until the heat dissipated and then go on to the next one. It took about 25 or 30 minutes, quite a bit of time. When I was done she hopped off the table, went home, and got everything ready for the trip.

Well, a week later, while still on vacation, she got a terrible headache and it was so bad her husband took her to the emergency room. They looked to see if there was an aneurism but they couldn't find anything, so they told her, "You will just have to get used to it." Can you imagine?

This was on a Wednesday, they flew home on Friday and she called and left a message on my answering machine to tell me what happened. By the time I was able to call her back she had been hospitalized and asked if I would come and do Healing Touch with her. When I walked in the room was all dark because she couldn't tolerate light, the light hurt her eyes and caused her headache to be worse. As I worked on her she feel asleep and was able to sleep most of the night.

So every night at 8:00 for the next ten days I went to the hospital and gave her a treatment. At the end of ten days her headache stopped and she was released. When she went in for a follow-up appointment she asked the doctor, "What do we do now?" and the doctor said, "What do you mean, what do we do now?" And she said, "How do you treat people from here on out?" and he said, "Only one percent of the people live through an aneurism and those are in nursing homes."

I have no idea what to make of the heat and the buzzing that I first felt. She said she had some sinus stuff going on, so I thought maybe her sinuses were a lot worse than she thought. About four years later she had something going on in her head and she went to the doctor but he didn't find anything. So she called me, she came in with a migraine, I treated her, it stopped about four hours later and it's never returned. That was about eight years ago and she always tells people I saved her life, but it was a power much stronger than mine.

In another case my daughter asked me if I would work on an elderly lady who had been helping her in her day care business. She had a stroke on the right side behind her ear and she was comatose. I worked on her for three days, just sending the energy into her body with the intention that the brain would heal; you know that intention is three-fourths of the thing. On the last day that I did a session with her, four hours after I was done, she woke up. She's in a wheelchair but her brain is in good shape, her mind is clear.

The next story is about a good friend of mine who lost her husband. She had been married before, had two children, she divorced that man because he was an alcoholic, then she married this wonderful man. She had had a very unhappy childhood, her parents weren't particularly parental, and she didn't really feel loved by them, but this man's parents treated her royally, so for the first time she had a family that she could go to.

They were married for three years then he died of cancer. So she called me one day and said, "My heart hurts so badly; will you help me?" And I said, "I will try." I had lost my husband when I was 43 so I knew what she was going through; I knew how that hurts.

So she came, I got her on the table and relaxed, and I started the session using Healing Touch interventions. As soon as I started all this energy was coming into the room and it just filled the entire room. I thought, "Wow, this is really neat!" I just kind of paid attention to that and I was grateful for it, and by the end of the session there was still all this energy in the room. It's a small room, 8x10 or something like that, so I backed up into the corner and I just stood there and waited with my hands out, holding the space, and gradually over four or five minutes that energy dissipated. I took her hand and said, "Are you okay?" And she said, "I didn't know you could bring the angels." And I said to myself, "What? I didn't know, either." That's what intention does. She said they were transparent, there were two of them, and the one took his hand and pointed it right at her heart and when he did that the pain dissipated. That was a divine moment, I'm telling you!

So she goes and tells a friend of hers and the friend comes and says, "I want to come and see the angels." I knew this woman, she had been on my table before, I wasn't particularly fond of her, and I said, "Well, you know, I can't promise anything, but if it's our intention we'll say a little prayer and see what happens."

So we went through our routine and everything and when I finished I said, "Are you okay?" and she said, "My mother died a year ago and she came to visit me and we had a wonderful talk." Isn't that great? I wish someone could have helped me with my grief, it's horrible, I thought I was going to die. I was ready to go, I could understand why so many couples die within a few months or a couple of years of each other, but we had five children and I thought, "Who would take care of those five children?" so maybe that's why I'm still here. This was in 1975 before all the grieving stuff came to the forefront and there was help for people.

What helped us as a family is that we talked a lot about him and just worked our way through it. The father of one of my piano students had died not long before this and she said something about not wanting to talk to her mother about it because it would make her mother cry. I said, "But that's exactly what you should do; what better person to cry with than your own mother?" So I followed my own advice, talk to these kids and find out what they're going through. One of my sons was very angry at his dad; grieving is a lot of things, and anger is one of them. Later in my career I did some work with a group that does weekend retreats for children who have lost parents or other family members. It was fascinating. I didn't do any work on the children, I just worked on the volunteers who were there, doing massage and Healing Touch.

My career has taken interesting twists and turns. I have a bachelor of science in music education so I taught, then after my husband died and we moved out West I became a financial planner. In 1990 I took a massage class and started working on friends and relatives, and then the next thing I know I'm working on my clients. So one week I'm investing money, the next week I'm over here doing massage and I thought, "This is really weird." After a couple of years of that I thought, "I think I'm supposed to be doing this other stuff. The financial planning is all right brained and the body work combines left and right brain which suits me much better."

There is a technique, a routine, that I created that I will share with you, which is simply having a person sit in a chair and concentrate on breathing out through their feet. I have them start the out-breath through the feet to get used to what that feels like, then I tell them to breathe out all of their mental, emotional, and physical concerns with each breath. It's amazing how much crap comes up out of the body to get rid of through the breathing and intention pattern. When the person feels complete with breathing out what they don't want, then I guide them through breathing in through the feet what they do want, such as more energy, strength, peace of mind, whatever.

I did this for my daughter and her husband one night. They had bought a new home and once they started to unpack they didn't stop until they practically dropped dead. My daughter was exhausted so I said, "Sit down, let me do this for you." I guided her through the routine, which took about fifteen or twenty minutes, and when we were done I thought she went upstairs and went to bed, but the next thing I knew she was running up and down the stairs. I said, "I thought you went to bed," and she said, "No, I'm just so full of energy now." I had her husband do the same breathing routine and it worked really well for him, too.

———————•◦•●●●•◦•———————

Knowing how to do energy work and massage has kept me healthy and has benefitted my family a great deal. I will sometimes use essential oils with my clients, particularly peppermint oil as an aura cleanser and to reduce pain, and also with family members. My daughter fell off her bike and hurt her rib and I used helichrysum for the pain. It's very expensive but very effective. Another time I used it was when a family member had a knee operation and when he was in the hospital they put him on a high toilet, he's a big man, the toilet fell over and he was black and blue, and I mean *black* from the accident. So I took him some helichrysum and mixed it with some carrier oil, rubbed it into the skin and told him to put it on again that night and the next morning. When I went to see him the next afternoon the bruising was practically all gone where typically it would have taken at least a couple of weeks to clear up, probably more.

Doing all the things that I do, massage, Healing Touch, Ortho-Bionics, essential oils, I love it and it has made a huge difference in my life. I am healthier than most people my age, eighty-four years old, and still going strong.

Marjorie
Master of Education
Teacher and High School Counselor, Retired
Theophostic Prayer Ministry
Reiki Practitioner
Healing Touch Practitioner

Introduction

Marjorie brought up two interesting aspects of using energy healing that deserve consideration for anyone who is doing the work. One of her questions was the appropriateness of having a complete stranger work so intimately with someone when they are very ill and close to death and may not be able to give clear consent in that very emotionally vulnerable state. The other is a related question about knowing when it isn't appropriate to do the work. She discusses this in the interview when she talks about her father's death and wonders if he was unwilling to receive because he was ready to die and somehow knew and was afraid that it would hold him back. Or maybe he thought it would hasten his death: there was no way to know what he was thinking. This issue highlights how important it is to get permission from the recipient when energy work is offered and not feel that we, as the practitioners, know what is best and proceed without consent.

Marjorie has taken classes in Healing Touch but is not a certified practitioner.

Interview

My background is kind of scattered, different jobs in different fields and lots of travel, but I eventually settled on teaching and have my Masters in Education. It was when I was working as a school counselor that I became interested in the different ways that energy is sent out from the human body. This was in the early years of scientific research in which Kirlian photography was used to photograph the energy field around plants and the human hand. I found that whole area fascinating as I always had a sense about the mysteries of life, the things that are not within our grasp and our understanding.

Three or four times my mother had dreams about people who soon after died, and in the dream there was a specific pattern. The pattern was that an animal had been killed, the person she was dreaming about was butchering it, and within a very short period of time this person would die in real life although there hadn't been any indications of ill health that she knew of. When her own parents were dying she knew before she got the phone calls that something was wrong and was already in the car on her way to where they lived. She just had that sense, that awareness, so I've always lived with it. Animals would come to her, coyotes would answer her call, things like that which don't make any logical sense, but I just accepted that something unexplainable was going on and it was real. Because of this background I didn't have any problem with the whole idea that there are energy fields around us and that they can be manipulated for our good or for our harm, so when I went to the energy healing classes, Therapeutic Touch and Healing Touch, it was just great fun to see how working with the energy can be done.

When I took the first Healing Touch class there was another student whom I worked with, a man in law enforcement; I was surprised that he was even in that setting. He was having a tremendous amount of guilt because he didn't want to take the treatments for the cancer that would prolong his life. He felt that he was letting down his ancestors, his parents and others who were deceased, his whole family lineage by not taking the treatments.

The intervention in that Level I class was simple, a clearing of the energy field, but in spite of that he had an experience that he described as having been given permission to die. He said that he saw those significant people, those family members who had gone before him, and they were giving him permission to do whatever he wanted to do. With that permission came freedom. He felt that his decision not to undergo any more treatments was honored and for the first time he didn't feel the weight of that guilt. This experience touched my heart, still touches it because it was so important to him. This was a man in a position of authority in his profession, had had to make many life and death decisions, yet here was an issue with his own dying and decisions about his life, and how emotional that was for him. I never saw him again, but that experience opened the way for him to have a peaceful death.

When my aunt was dying I showed her daughter and granddaughter how to do a Healing Touch intervention to help sooth and calm her. She was in a coma but appeared to be struggling, so showing them how to do this allowed them to do something to help instead of feeling completely helpless.

The next time I was with someone who was dying was with my father. The nurses had come in to check on him and they said that it would be several hours before he died, maybe not until the next day. When I was with him I was praying with him, he'd had a stroke so he couldn't speak, but he was aware because when I would speak to him he would look at me and he was aware of what I was saying. That afternoon he was looking out the window, looking away from me, when I started to do a Healing Touch technique. I still to this day do not know if he saw the motion or he felt it, but he looked at me and his expression was like, "What are you doing? No, I don't give you permission to do that, stop," so I stopped. That's an uneasy memory for me because I could have asked him permission, he was aware, but it's almost as if I was being sneaky or underhanded about it, wanting to help him die but not able to say that.

The nurse came in right after that to say she was going to clean up my father and asked that I leave the room for a few minutes, so I stepped out and within just a few minutes of my leaving he died. At the meal after Dad's funeral several of us were talking, one of whom is a nurse, and the conversation was about how common it is for a person to die when everybody has left the room, whereas some people will hang on until a particular event, like a visit from a particular person, or a birthday or graduation. Both my sister and I were feeling guilty that we had left him because we had been told that it would be some time before he died, but knowing that this often happens, and remembering that he didn't want any energy healing, I think he wanted to die then with no one and nothing to hold him back. But before I left the room I was able to tell him that I loved him, tell him all the things that I wanted to, so that was good.

With my mom, who died less than a week before her 100th birthday, the experience was different. Over the last few years of her life she had recovered from cancer, recovered from strokes, had suffered severe bladder infections, and was suffering from dementia. One day I got a call from the assisted living center she was in and was told that she wasn't responding to the staff and they wanted her to get medical treatment. My sister and I arranged for her to be taken to the hospital and were told that she had only a few days left to live. While we were deciding what environment she would want to be in for her passing, and thinking that we would have her taken back to her room in assisted living and call in hospice, she remained in the hospital.

I have a friend, Mary, who worked with hospice, and her main function is to sing to people who are terminal, often singing to them as they are dying, whatever kind of music they want. She heard that my mother was in the hospital and that she was dying, so she came and sang different religious songs that my mother would have known. My mother didn't seem to be responding although she was trying to talk. Unfortunately, we hadn't brought her teeth so I couldn't understand most of what she was saying.

One of the songs that Mary sang is called "The Divine Mercy Prayer," and I later learned that this is a prayer that is often said to help people who are dying to have a peaceful death. I was uneasy about doing any energy healing because of my experience with my dad and the conflicting emotions that one may have about their own family members. I wanted to give her healing energy, but it also felt as if maybe I was hastening her death because she had been through so much already and I really didn't want her to have to go through any more.

I found that I didn't want to touch her, feeling that my touch would hold her back, that maybe it would ground her into this life or hold her back and I didn't want to do that if that wasn't what she wanted. My sister and I both agreed that we did not want her to be bedridden; it would have been horrible for her to be paralyzed or bedridden or unable to communicate. She was already experiencing dementia, and there were some things that were happening that were heart breaking. Even before this there would be times when she would be frightened and disoriented, wouldn't know how to find the dining room when she left her room. This is a person who graduated from college magna cum laud, spoke four different languages, just extremely bright and a leader in all kinds of ways, but needed reassurance that somebody would be there for her.

So I think that it was important for her not to die alone, that she would hear my voice and my friend's voice in those last hours. I did energy healing but I didn't touch her, just did gentle movements above her and around her heart. She didn't seem to be responding to me, but Mary told me later that that was exactly what she needed. I trust her observations because she has been at a number of deaths through hospice. So I did the energy healing, together we sang the song three or four times, and when we got to the very end my mother had died. Mary said that in all of her experiences with people dying this was the most peaceful death she had witnessed. Some people are struggling so hard, physically struggling, trying to catch another breath, and she said that as she was singing she could see my mother's breathing being more and more calm. There would be a breath, but it was so peaceful that there was not a specific breath of death, it was just gentle until there was no breath at all. Mary said that as she was watching my mother before she died it looked as if she were looking at something outside of us that was present to her but that we couldn't see.

I haven't had any afterlife communication from my mother, although my sister, who doesn't really believe in such things, had her daughter come to her in a dream. My sister has a very difficult time dealing with the fact that she wasn't able to be with her daughter when she died, but she came to her in a dream in which she let her mother know that she was alright, that she was in a good place, and it was alright that she wasn't there at the time of her death. When my sister remembers the dream she is very comforted, but when she remembers the event as it happened she's not.

So you see that I felt conflicted using Healing Touch with my parents, and with my friends and clients I never do energy healing without also using prayer. There is a power beyond what I can understand, so for people who may be conflicted because of their religious beliefs it helps to have prayer as part of the sessions. There are two worlds that we are dealing with, this one and the spiritual world, so I work with both.

I also do a counseling process called Theophostic Prayer Ministry. This comes from a Christian background so it is particularly helpful for people who have a religious orientation and believe in God or a higher power. It is a way to deal with events from the past that one is still carrying around in their psyche and causing sadness, or reactions to events in the present that are so over-reactive that it doesn't make sense to them. Together we pray that Jesus show them the truth of the situations and heal them from the false conclusions that were drawn from them.

When I am working with someone in grief I may use the Theophostic process because of the unfinished business they are still carrying around with them, their fears, and their uncharacteristic reactions which they don't understand and are embarrassed about. One woman I worked with dreaded living alone for the first time in her life; she was dealing well with the loss of her husband except for this fear of being alone. It was disrupting her life but because of the work she was able to build her self-confidence and feel more emotionally balanced. An interesting consequence was her ability to deal with some of her more difficult relatives.

I am always so humbled that people trust me enough to come to me with the most vulnerable aspects of themselves: I feel very honored by that. But this brings me to some concerns that I have about offering

Healing Touch to people whom you don't know and they don't know you, particularly when they are in the process of dying.

The problem with the energy as a person is dying is that it becomes so mixed up because the people around the patient are in such an emotionally heightened state, are in such distress, there is so much fear and confusion, so it's hard for me to imagine that the dying person would consent to receiving anything more unless you already had a relationship established with them. If not, how would you explain it to them in terms that were compatible with their religious and cultural beliefs so that you weren't inappropriately crossing boundaries? What if you were the patient who felt uncomfortable with the person offering it to you, or you had an instinctive dislike of that person? If you or I were in the hospital somewhere and asked for Healing Touch, how would that request be interpreted? If the staff or volunteers were trained in the Healing Touch, with capital H and capital T, they would know what we were asking for, but otherwise how would a request for Healing Touch/healing touch be understood? When you and I think about the people in our own Healing Touch community, are there people that you would not want in your space, not want them to see you and work with you at your most vulnerable time? These are the questions that I have about when to offer it, when it is an appropriate thing to do and when it isn't.

What do I want to say about death? I was miraculously saved from a serious automobile accident, so I believe in Divine intervention, but that doesn't mean I don't fear death because I do. I think the fear is a natural human condition and that is probably a good thing because maybe it prompts us to live a kinder, nicer life than we would otherwise. It would be helpful to have more education about what happens to our bodies during the death process because a lot of us are afraid of what will happen; it certainly helped me when my father was dying and the nurse came in and talked to me about it. She said that as the body shuts down the patient doesn't experience thirst. Earlier I might have thought that would be the worst thing in the world, to stop liquids because it's so painful, but it turns out that's not true. Learning more about the process made a difference in how I want to die, and I put in my Advanced Medical Directive to withhold food and liquids at a certain point because I don't want to exist for months and months, or even days and days when it is my time to go.

Jean
Registered Nurse
Reiki Master
Healing Touch Board Certified Practitioner (National Commission
for Certifying Agencies designation)
Healing Touch Board Certified Instructor

Introduction

Jean is a nurse whose career has included traditional nursing early on but then transitioned into many administrative and teaching positions. In most of these positions there was, and is, no opportunity to formally use Healing Touch, but many co-workers who know that she does this work and that she has a home-based private holistic practice will ask about it. She is a Healing Touch Certified Practitioner and a Healing Touch Certified Instructor. The Veterans Administration has a mandate to incorporate holistic practices into the care they offer patients, with Healing Touch being one of them. Jean is the instructor for those classes in her city of residence.

Interview

I've been a nurse for fifty years, and the nursing that I was taught had an element of hands-on care. We did back rubs, we sat and took time listening to the patients, and we were taught to look at body language. There's no time for that anymore. The advantage of being able to do Healing Touch, when there's time to do it, is that any time you do Healing Touch it's not depleting, it's energizing, we're just working in the energy field. We could be doing more of that in the hospital, in our nursing practices, and if we did nurses would be more energized, they would have more stamina, they would have more job satisfaction.

I learned about Therapeutic Touch and Healing Touch in a workshop for nurses that I was invited to attend by a nurse friend. I had already learned Reiki, I was a Reiki Master, but when I found out that Healing Touch is a program that came out of the body of nursing I thought, "Oh, my gosh. Here is something that's evidence based, it comes out of nursing, it's got a Western medicine model to it," so I just embraced it and took the first class that was offered. I was working in public health at that time and I really missed the one-on-one contact, so being able to do Healing Touch sessions in my private practice kind of met that need. In comparison to Reiki, I found that Healing Touch gives so much more freedom to be able to make an assessment and determine, almost minute by minute, how you are going to work with the energy field. It's all the same energy but with Healing Touch I was able to use a lot more of my nursing skills, even though we don't diagnose, which is beyond our scope of practice, but to at least help me intuitively to know what was going on and pay attention and not just do something by rote. Every client is different and the program gives the opportunity for the practitioner to tailor it to that individual. At the end of the session we can discuss with them things they can do to enhance their healing, so there is that teaching part that I like and had done for so long.

A nice thing about Healing Touch is that while we're dealing with the biofield, the human energy field, we still use Western medicine protocol as far as assessment, summary, observation, referral, and future planning, with the intention to support and facilitate mental, emotional, and spiritual health. Because of advancements in medicine we have all these specialists but nobody puts us back together, whereas with Healing Touch we are looking at the whole person, looking at everything that is going on, not just the physical.

I've done work with patients who have physical symptoms that no one has been able to solve, and when we're able to go deeper and look at the energy system and where it's compromised, the things that come out of that can be a major key to recovery. I had a young woman who had so many problems with her female system, and after many months of working with her she was able to relate that she had been physically abused. Once she was able to integrate all of that and share it, she healed. In spite of all the tests and appointments and surgeries it didn't go away, we had to go to a different level for healing to occur. She signed releases so that her physician and I could keep each other informed of what we were doing, and it proved to be a very productive relationship for all involved.

We don't have time in the Western medical model for our physicians and health care workers to explore the underlying causes of conditions that won't heal, to go back into a person's history and look at the energetics of traumas that the body still holds, so if they would work with us and we could support each other we would have a truly integrative medical system. One day I was doing a session with a patient in the hospital and the doctor waited outside the door until we were finished. When he came in he said, "I wish you could be here every day." What a wonderful acknowledgement of the benefits of the work, and as practitioners we also wish we could be there everyday.

Energy healing remains a mystery to a lot of people, others may never have heard of it or may simply dismiss it. We want people to understand that it's something that we're taught to do with our hands in a heart-centered manner, that we don't diagnose, we are trained to follow the energy, and the whole purpose of Healing Touch is to clear and to balance the energy field so that the individual's physiology, their physical, mental, and spiritual systems can do what they are designed to do so there is greater potential for healing. There are research studies that show the benefits of energy healing, in other words it is an evidence based practice, and more research is being done all the time.

The biggest issue is that there is no funding to create paid positions so we have to rely on volunteers at their convenience. We do have one free clinic a month at a local hospital for anyone to come for sessions, including hospital staff. Just this week I worked with a woman who had plantar fasciitis who was in such pain, and by the time she got off the table the pain was gone. She was also having neck pain, so I had her turn over onto her stomach and did a back technique because it wasn't just her neck that needed the work, it was also her back. Sometimes the staff members will come for a session as they are leaving work, others will come back for the energy boost and the opportunity to have deep relaxation. If our health insurance would cover once-a-month visits for preventive health care, be it acupuncture, massage, Healing Touch, Reiki, whatever, people would be healthier; it's just a no brainer.

I have always been interested in the spiritual aspects of things, and very interested in self-care and self-healing. That is a big part of my life, part of my purpose.

In the Healing Touch Program™ there is an emphasis and an expectation that we will do self-care, have a spiritual practice, continue to grow and evolve, and to always let go of ego, let go of the outcome. It's been a great thing. I think it has held my feet to the fire to continue my own spiritual practice, my own self-care, to be a role model. I think without that it's just too easy to let some of that slip away and get a little bit lazy about it.

Professionally, I would have to say that wherever I have worked, the fact that I can be centered and grounded, and compassionate and loving, has enabled me to get through any kind of crisis in a work situation. Even in my current position we've had some things come up that everybody was in an uproar about, and I can usually put something into words that makes sense and gets everybody back to being centered and grounded again. It's helpful for any work situation I've been in, it's made a big difference. Once you are trained in energy healing and practice it, it becomes a part of who you are. I had somebody call me today who was in a twit about something and instead of getting entrained by her energy I just said, "Okay, stop, I'd like you to breathe." And she said, "I know that, but I forget." Simple things like that, but not so simple, like what happened with my son.

My son was trekking in the Himalayas and he contracted a very nasty eye infection. By the time he got to a medical facility they took one look at him, immediately put him in a taxi to the airport, and flew him to a hospital in Singapore where the doctors told him he was probably going to lose his eye.

So he called me, I was at a conference, but the minute I got off the phone I started working with him long distance. I forgot to even ask him which eye it was, but the minute I closed my eyes I knew exactly which eye it was, it was very obvious. Every spare moment I got I worked on him. He was finally discharged and the medical staff there said it was a miracle that he didn't lose his eye. He did end up doing a corneal transplant, but he didn't lose his eye. Physics says that distance makes no difference in the ability for energy to be transmitted and affect the intended target, so I have no doubt that distance healing works.

When I am doing distance healing for a client I have them set time aside if they can, and I call them and will do the session with them while they are listening in. I like doing distance healing because I'm not distracted by the connection we have that could skew my thoughts. I will put garments on the treatment table and adjust them to represent the person I am working on, state my intention for the session, and ask to be shown the person's energy field. Once I feel the connection I proceed just as if they were there in person. I actually think I'm more effective when I do distance work just because I'm totally relying on my connection to spirit, my connection to that person's biofield.

There is very little conversation during the process, but at least they feel like they're connected and we can give each other feedback and ask questions. At the end I will give them a little recap about what I sensed, ask how they are feeling, if they experience any changes, and answer any questions they may have. Then I chart the session just as if they were here in my treatment room.

I have a story about the power of intention. When I was teaching and working with students doing hospital rotations, one of the gals was a Certified Nursing Assistant (CNA) working in the intensive care unit, and one of her patients was a woman who was dying. In the Healing Touch advanced training there is a technique taught that helps people transition into a more peaceful death, so she thought,

"I'll go in and do this technique on this lady because she's in a coma and is on her way out."

The CNA went into the room to do an assessment and something stopped her. She sensed that this woman was not giving her permission to work in her field and it kind of baffled her. So she went home and when she came back the next day the woman had come out of her coma; she was not ready to die. So it was a real lesson for this student: we don't go in with the intention that we're going to help somebody cross over, we go in to make them comfortable and let them be at peace for whatever the outcome is. But she said it was so profound, she was just stopped, literally stopped in her tracks and knew that this woman did not want her to do the process she had intended to do and she couldn't imagine why. The next day she found out why – the woman was not ready to go.

So we have to be careful about our intention, careful about getting our ego out of the way and feeling that we know what is best for the person or what the person may want if they can't tell us. I've been called into the hospital quite a few times to work with someone, several of them were elderly, but one that I remember in particular was a young man who had been in a horrible automobile accident. The intention was not to help him have a peaceful death but to ease the pain and anxiety and allow whatever the outcome from the accident would be. The family was in the room and it gave them so much peace to palpably and visually see the young man relaxing and looking more comfortable. For this to happen, for this to possibly be the last vision of their loved one, I think this is a gift to the patient and the family.

Being able to help others is also a gift for the practitioner. I was able to help my mom after her open heart surgery. She was a really good candidate, the prognosis was good, but she apparently had another heart attack during surgery so she did not do well afterwards. They had her sedated, she was on a ventilator, and she never recovered. Because of the sedation and the tube she was not able to talk to me, but I had done years and years of Healing Touch on her so I knew that she recognized my energetic touch, and just the fact that I could be with her and do Healing Touch was such a blessing for both of us. I was able to be with her in an intimate way and not feel helpless to do anything.

What I observed as I was working on her was relaxation, her face relaxing, her breathing slowing down, just a lot more peacefulness. Try to imagine what it's like to be having a tube breathe for you, a machine breathe for you, and not being able to talk and not being fully conscious, how frightening that must be. It was very noticeable how calming the Healing Touch was. The calming and relaxation is a typical response to the work. I did Healing Touch with an American Buddhist monk who had been diagnosed with parotid gland cancer and we worked together for his healing before his surgery. He was able to go into a deep state of meditation and relaxation during the session. The outcome was that when he went in for the surgery they did not find the tumor that had been seen on the MRI.

Energy work isn't just for physical healing. I was working on a woman at a free Healing Touch clinic and when I was finished I asked the man with her if he would like to experience it. At first he said no, he had just come to support his friend, but eventually he did get on the table. I sensed that there was something not quite right about his energy, and when I scanned his energy field it was very hard to discern it because it was so close to his body, almost immeasurable. He shared that he had been chronically depressed. I started seeing him weekly and then monthly and his depression gradually resolved. I also made the appropriate referrals to other health professionals. He received some good care and support, but I felt that it was the Healing Touch that put all the pieces together; physical, emotional, and spiritual.

It is so rewarding for me to see someone's health improve, and the great thing is that Healing Touch can be learned by anyone and can be used on yourself or on others. There is a course of study leading to certification for those who want to become practitioners. You don't need any tools, all you need is your hands and your heart. The founder of the program, Janet Mentgen, said that her goal, her vision, was to have someone in every home across the world know how to do Healing Touch.

Wouldn't that be nice? How many parents and grandparents

would love to have something as simple as that to ease the pain from the accidents that kids have, and for the adults as well? When I was first learning Healing Touch, one of the first times I had the courage to use it in public was at a retreat. We had been outside taking a break and were getting ready to go back in and reassemble when a young man in front of me tripped on the curb and twisted his ankle. He sat down and was obviously in agony, so I came over to him and I said, "I know something, Healing Touch, and if you're willing I'd like to see if I could work on that." I sat down on the curb next to him and did a couple of techniques to ease the pain and I could see the swelling going down. He was able to get up and walk back in, and when I checked with him later he said he had a little bit of pain but that was all.

Whether it's for physical pain, emotional pain, helping with major life transitions including moving from life into death, Healing Touch can help. It's a gift for me to be able to be a part of facilitating the changes, and doing Healing Touch for somebody who is in transition feels very sacred, very intimate. The bond that is created with somebody when you're sharing that space with them is a privilege.

In working with the dying I have been able to teach relatives how to do some techniques so that they feel much more a part of the process, to not feel so helpless like there's nothing they can do except stand by and watch. By introducing Healing Touch into the dying process it allows everybody around that person to feel like there's some help for that person. I always invite people to stay in the room when I do a session, and even people who aren't familiar with energy work pick up on the energy, how the feeling in the room changes. I often do sessions on the people who are close to the person who is dying because it helps them deal with the loss.

One of the comments I'd like to make about death in general is that other cultures have a whole different view of death, they have more openness about it, they have rituals, they accept it as part of the life cycle, but here in this country we fight it tooth and nail. People don't want to let go, relatives don't want to let people go, and nobody wants to talk about it, which leaves the dying person in quite a predicament. Being able to face what is happening allows for open communication, which makes such a difference at the end of a person's life. The one who is dying is able to express him or herself, and those who are left behind can be more at peace because of the conversations that were had and the thoughts and emotions that were expressed. So having Healing Touch to do in the transition process certainly helps open up the dialogue about what's best for the person, what's for their highest good, allowing them to transition in a dignified way.

Annie
Bachelor of Science in Nursing
Certified Healing Touch Practitioner

Introduction

The role that death and personal injury has played in Annie's life were strong influences in her discovery of Healing Touch, and her desire to use it professionally was the deciding factor in completing the program through certification. She is currently retired from nursing but has a private healing practice.

Interview

My father was a physician, my mother was a nurse, and I think it was expected that I would become a nurse too, that I would do something where I was helping people. Many of my friends had degrees that didn't lead to jobs once they were out of school, but once you graduate with nurses training you can get a job right away, so it was a reasonable thing for me to do.

For much of my career I was a public health nurse, but even in my hospital nursing I had never seen anybody die, I'd never been around a dead body, so the death of my husband was my first direct experience with death. Then my father died, my mother died, and my beloved dog of twelve and half years died. The dog is the only one I did Healing Touch on because I didn't know about it before then.

My husband died of mesothelioma seventeen months after he had been diagnosed. It extended up his neck and into his brain, and he knew he was losing function and his thinking capacities. He was very healthy otherwise, incredibly fit, very muscular and strong, just a very active, very smart person. For a long time he fought very hard to stay alive because he didn't believe in an afterlife, but he wasn't open to hearing about energy healing from my sister so that wasn't any part of his treatment. Then one day he wouldn't eat and I said, "But you have to eat," and he said, "Why, why do I have to eat? I'm done. I don't want you to feed me and I don't want you to give me any water at all, I'm done."

As a nurse that's really hard to hear, but I had to respect that he had been fighting for a long time and he was tired. He did not want to talk about death, did not want to talk about anything like that, so I had to respect it. The next day he did not get out of bed and when I offered him food and water he did not want it. He did agree to let me keep his mouth hydrated, and he did have some pain pills from hospice, but by refusing to eat or drink he basically committed suicide. It was hard to watch, but I knew he was doing it his way so I loved and supported him and did what I could for him.

He stopped eating on a Monday and on that Friday a friend came and got me and said I had to go to the funeral home to make arrangements. I hadn't done anything prior to that because of his refusal to talk about death. When I returned from the funeral home my sister was at the house and we went into his bedroom to reposition him and that's when he died.

It was interesting because we were repositioning him and he was sitting up, and all of a sudden he stopped breathing. Even though you know it's coming it was shocking. Then he opened his eyes and he looked at me, but then he looked beyond me and he got this most glorious look in his eyes. He was instantly so happy, I could see it in his eyes, it was just a wonderful moment. Then he closed his eyes, he hadn't been breathing, and slowly his energy transitioned out. I was so happy for him because I knew that he learned he wasn't alone, that he was going to make his transition just fine. That was glorious, and it was a very good lesson and comforting for me to see.

The second death that I was there for was my father's. He fell in the basement and suffered a spiral fracture to the femur. He had a history of heart disease and had been on a blood thinner for years, so they couldn't do surgery unless they gave him something that would allow the blood to clot so he wouldn't bleed to death during the operation.

He did not want surgery, but my mother and brother overruled him so they started giving him the drug. I could not convince my mom to let him be, to let him do it his way.

As a physician he knew that his heart was bad enough that by being immobilized he would probably end up in a nursing home or he would get pneumonia and die anyway, and he didn't want to go through the surgery and the recovery when he knew there was little chance of a long, good life after that. He just wanted to be left alone to die, that's what he wanted, that was his choice, but since other people were making a different choice for him he took matters into his own hands. It was awful to see what he went through and I tried very hard to get them to stop doing things against his wishes. I finally was going to call in a specialist doctor that I knew, a friend of mine who did a lot of end-of-life care who could talk to them, but before I could do that he died.

You know those little triangle bars above a hospital bed? Well, he was doing chin-ups with those, trying very hard to rupture his heart, trying to overdo his heart, and he eventually did, he ruptured the mitral valve and died. Prior to this they had given him forty-three bags of the coagulant medication and his chemistries did not change a bit. It was an interesting lesson for me because it appeared that no matter what anybody else did his determination to die was the overriding factor. It was hard to see the way he did it, but he did the best he could in the circumstances he had: he knew what he wanted and he'd been there, done that, seen a lot of patients, and he didn't want to go down that road.

Before he died he was talking with people beyond the veil, he was seeing many people beyond the veil, so I knew he was connected, I knew he would be okay, it was just a matter of timing, and he managed to die when the people who objected the most were out of the room.

My mom's death was different and I don't think I learned anything from it. She was living in a retirement home, very busy and active, when she got pneumonia. In the hospital she got the bacterial infection C. difficile, which was not diagnosed correctly, and they sent her to a nursing home. When I went to visit her she was worse so I got her taken to the hospital immediately, but by then it was too late and she was going into organ failure. The doctor ordered morphine for her and it may have been a heavy enough dose to help her on her way. She had some wonderful hallucinations, and I don't know how much was the medication or how much was actually coming through in spirit. There wasn't anything I could do for her, but at least I was there supporting her and supporting my sisters.

With my dog I was able to do several Healing Touch techniques that helped with the pain in his back. I knew he was starting to fail, but one day he just couldn't get up and I could tell he was ready to go. It was very interesting to watch him, he just kind of seemed to have the attitude that dying was no big deal. I took him to his favorite fishing spot and the vet met us there, he gave him medicine and he was gone. Then about twenty seconds later we're sitting here in this beautiful spot at a picnic table, all of a sudden this huge rain and dust storm hit us – boom, hit us for about thirty seconds – and then it was gone. It blew everything over, it got us covered with dust, and then it was gone. I'm sure that was him telling us he had made a successful transition. So three out of four of my closest deaths have taught me wonderful things and it's all about how powerful we are, that we create how our life is and when and how we're going to go, and who will be there. From what I've seen, and the messages that have come through psychics, it seems that people can plan when they die or they can take advantage of something that comes up, like my nephew apparently did.

My nephew was born with a heart problem and ended up having surgery. At some point he was oxygen deprived so he had some neurological deficits and found it difficult to function in the world. At the next channeling session I went to I asked to talk to him and asked him what happened. He said: "I was thirty-two years old and I realized I was still a burden to my family, my parents were getting older, and I just felt like a burden. So I got this cold and I let it take me; instead of just getting over the cold I let it lead to shutting down my organ systems and I died. That was my choice, that I let that happen, and I'm much happier now." It seems that he had not planned when to die but instead took an opportunity to leave.

The whole idea of having this much control over our own death was something that my dad kind of taught me. I remember that he was talking about two of his patients and the will to live, which could be described as the ability to command your own body. One patient had recurring bouts of cancer, seven different cancers, and survived. Another patient who was perfectly healthy had a very small problem, nothing serious like cancer or pneumonia, and died. So it seems that it was much like my nephew who wanted to go and allowed something small to take him out.

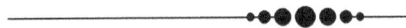

I may never have found and practiced energy healing if my husband had lived. I would have continued to be very physically based, practiced very physically based medicine because he would have ridiculed energy medicine. He was very scientifically oriented, and if he didn't believe there is an afterlife, obviously he didn't believe in anything spiritual, so if I had gone in that direction it would have been a battle, we might have gotten divorced. He didn't want to go down the spiritual path, he wasn't spiritual at all, but I wanted to explore the spiritual; my illnesses and accident led me there.

Before my first health crisis I was working in a job I didn't like, I wanted to quit, but the paycheck was good so I stayed, but then I got breast cancer. My body knew what to do even though I didn't, or wouldn't, and it got me out of the situation. The cancer didn't kill me, it kind of got me to a spiritual place where I said, "God, I give up," and the next week I had a 104 fever that lasted a week and that cured my cancer.

Then I fell down the stairs and broke my neck, but I still wasn't quite into the spiritual thing, still some resistance. After that, when I was vacationing in Hawaii, I had a total bowel obstruction and right before going under the knife I said, "Okay, God, do not send me back unless you help me figure out what I am going to do for the rest of my life because I haven't figured it out yet."

So I woke up and it was, "Okay, you're going to have to show me, I'm still here." Soon after that I went to a Wellness Festival and was directed to go to a brown bag presentation, and it was about Healing Touch. As soon as I heard about it I said, "Yes, this is it. I'm supposed to continue my nursing, helping, but I can do it without sticking pins and needles in people, I can do it in a way that is much more powerful than medicine will ever be, and in a way that daily increases my spiritual connection, that gives me support for everything that is going on."

I want to work with people who are wanting to open up and connect, and my goal with them is self-empowerment, spiritual opening, awareness of the energy in and around them, and increased ability to communicate with their guides. I really feel strongly that that's one of my best gifts, to help people connect.

One of my long-term clients was a lady with macular degeneration, she was blind in one eye. She was told that she would never see again out of that eye, we started working together, and through the many sessions that we had I talked to her about energy and helped her understand about thought patterns and maybe symbolically what it was she didn't want to see. We spent time doing a life review and we tried to do some past lives, too. Now, after about two years of working together, she has color vision and acuity in the outside part of her eye, and in the middle where it had been just gray she is starting to see shapes and colors.

Along with Healing Touch and the other things I mentioned, I asked her to practice looking out the window at something, using her good eye, and then to look straight at it with her bad eye and imagine that she is seeing it clearly through that eye. She needed to reactivate her brain, and even though she had to imagine it, it did reactivate the brain and I think that was a very powerful thing for her to have done for herself between our Healing Touch sessions. She's big into gratitude so we worked with affirmations, too. She's seeing, it's not black any more, she never went to a doctor because she's stubborn and I couldn't get her to go, but she did the work, she's healing herself, and she's living proof of what is possible.

Another case that stands out for me is one that illustrates the pain relief that Healing Touch can bring about. I was on duty at the hospital and I was asked to see this lady because she was in extreme pain from shoulder surgery and it wasn't time for her medication. I walked in the door and I could feel that her pain field was so huge that it was out the door. So I just started talking to her and put my hand on the edge of the pain field and I could feel it slowly collapse. It took me about twenty minutes to clear it, and when I got in close enough I engaged her and asked her to start talking about herself. By then I was close enough to her to be able to collapse the pain field around her and we started to talk and laugh because she was pain free and okay to wait until her next pain pill. That was very dramatic, going from totally wigged out to laughing and relaxed, sitting up and comfortable. So yes, Healing Touch works to reduce or eliminate pain, it works very well.

Physical pain isn't the only pain that Healing Touch helps ease. When I was doing the hundred sessions required for certification I asked a neighbor if she would be interested in receiving a session and she said yes. She was suffering from terrible depression and just as I laid hands on her, all of a sudden this big black gargoyle came up out of her chest and just flew at me. I called for spiritual help immediately, my guides came and grabbed it and I said, "Please take it and turn it into love because I don't know what to do with it." I finished the treatment and decided not to tell her about it because she wasn't into energy and such things, I just asked her how she was feeling. She said, "I feel much lighter." Since then I have seen attachments and thought forms that linger in a person's energy field, and energy medicine can help get rid of those even if they are many years old.

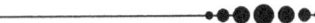

So I just want to say that learning Healing Touch and other forms of energy healing has empowered me to know that I can help people without hurting them, and without poisoning them with medications. When family members and friends see the relief that energy work can bring to their loved one they are open to learning it so they can be of help. For me, I benefit physically, emotionally, spiritually, and mentally every time I step into the healing energy. For nursing staff who receive Healing Touch it is wonderful for stress reduction and renewal. Being cared for is such a gift when you have been caring for others day after day.

What I want to say about death is that being with someone who is dying is a wonderful experience; not only can you be so supportive of them, and be quiet and listen and be there for them, but it's a great teaching experience for you. It showed me what a gift it was, and I came to feel that it was a graduation, that dying is graduation. It's not to be feared, it's a wonderful event. I would say to people to just be present at the end, be present and allow what happens to happen, and know that it's all in your highest good.

Carol
Licensed Clinical Professional Counselor
Healing Touch Practitioner

Introduction

At the time of our interview Carol had been in private practice for thirty-three years as a Licensed Clinical Professional Counselor (LCPC). She has a separate healing practice as a Healing Touch Practitioner, volunteers at a monthly Healing Touch free clinic at a local hospital, and for the past three years coordinated the offering of Healing Touch at an annual cancer retreat for women.

Interview

I have long been interested in people's life experiences and the many modalities of insight, care, and soothing that can be offered to them. My earliest memory is being eight and coming home from Catholic mass and saying to myself, "Our bodies are too incredible to only live once; there must be other stuff that happens to us." I think that was the beginning of having a clarity and a different path at a very young age, so I have branched out and sought many different modalities and teachings throughout my lifetime.

Healing Touch came to me through my neighbor, my mentor, my good friend Jean (see Jean's interview). When I experienced Healing Touch I was deeply drawn to the ease of doing it, but also drawn into the protocol around it that created a formal foundation and baseline with pre-and post-testing, and the ways through the protocol that we can check to see if we are impacting and making a change for people. That level of professionalism added to my draw to it. Any time I am exposed to any kind of energy healing work I am so aware of the depth of the energy, the intuitiveness, the power, the spirituality, and every time I have that experience it makes me want to have more.

I experienced a couple of Healing Touch sessions with Jean, then I took Level I training and at that point I was just hooked and very passionate about it and just kept going through the levels. I was amazed yet not surprised at the results and the impact that Healing Touch has on people's energy, their bodies and their attitude, and their hearts and their souls.

As a licensed counselor I am required to take CEUs and I would come home exhausted physically, mentally, and intellectually. I had learned copious amounts but I was tired, physically tired more than anything else, but also tired of just sitting and listening, thinking, "I'm going to finish getting through this," and I do it with grace but I'm aware that I am tired.

But the difference between that kind of workshop and a Healing Touch workshop, well, even though we're there Friday night until 9:00 or 9:30, all day Saturday, Saturday night, all day Sunday, I come out of there popping, like little popcorn kernels, full of energy, ready to go, not tired, not exhausted, not spent, just totally energized. I wasn't anticipating that and didn't even think about the difference until about halfway through the workshop that I realized, "I'm not tired, wow!" One of the ways I would describe energy work is that it is expansive, it's in cadence, it's in resonance with the inner part of my spirituality, it balances and rebalances me in a way that is totally energetic. It has become an irreplaceable part of my life.

The people whom I have worked with at end of life have been personal friends, not clients. I have long been drawn to the crossing over, the dying process, probably partially because I lived with my grandparents and my grandfather died when I was just short of twenty, and my father died when I was nineteen. My father died in a hospital, but I woke up, probably when he crossed over, because my mother and I remember that we were both awake when the call came from the hospital that he had died. So I think that my experience of bearing witness to my father's death opened me to not having any fear or apprehension, but having an inquisitive nature about death, being drawn to it rather than being repelled by it.

One person whom I worked with at end of life was a very near and dear colleague of mine; I'll call him Paul. Paul introduced me to my husband and we have been married for over twenty years.

Paul was a phenomenally spiritual person but not very religious. When I told him that I was learning Healing Touch I asked if he would be willing to let me work on him. He said okay, not very enthusiastically I might add, and by that time his ALS had progressed to the point where he was confined to a wheelchair and deteriorating physically. I continued to do Healing Touch with him over the following months, probably twelve times in all, and the last session was in the early evening the day before he died. Both my husband and I were there as we were his "A Team."

At the end he was in a semi-induced medical coma with a PIC line and a lot of sedation because he was having trouble breathing. I crawled up on the bed with him, checked his chakras, and the only chakra that was open was his crown chakra. I did the intervention with him that we were taught that helps people who are in major life transitions, including transitioning from life into death, and as I did that the energy in the room, the emotional connection, was absolutely profound and tangible. I was teary, his wife would poke her head in periodically and just give me a nod, and as the session progressed his breathing slowed to a beautiful calm cadence. It was not always smooth, even though he was in that semi-induced coma, but as the session progressed his breathing became much more evenly cadenced and I watched a little bit of color come into his face and his muscles relaxed. I had a very deep sense that I was surrounded by a variety of spiritual beings and guides.

His non-verbal, spiritual, energetic connection during that final Healing Touch session was the most profound connection; it was almost as if the space between us went away, wasn't visible, wasn't present, that there was a blending, a braiding, an integrating. I had a sense of him being tethered, but not tethered to the earth, tethered to the heavens, to what was to come out there. I felt the deepest sense of honor to be a part of that process, that I was bearing witness to something bigger than the universe itself. It was exquisite, it was humbling, it was tender-hearted, it was gently energetic, and I felt incredibly grounded before, during, and after the session. There was no fear, I didn't sense any fear in Paul's body as his muscles relaxed even more during the session. I was just aware that he kind of melted; it was absolutely exquisite. So being a part of his last hours was an incredible gift for which I will be eternally grateful.

Another person that I was privileged to work with right before her death was my surrogate mother, I'll call her Bess. She was a very sweet woman who was in my life for almost twenty years and she allowed me to do Healing Touch on her many times; I think she was fascinated with it. She was 92 years old at the time of her death.

Bess had fallen, and when I went to see her she was bedridden and in and out of a very light coma. She would open her eyes and recognize people, but she had macular degeneration so her eyesight was very poor. I gave her a Healing Touch treatment on two different days, and when I checked her chakras prior to the second treatment the only chakra that was open was her crown chakra, which had also been the case with Paul. I thought to myself, "Of course, that makes sense, she doesn't need any energy going anywhere except up to the universe where she's headed." And watching, again, the breathing slowing and becoming very even, the furrow leave her face, the little muscles by her mouth soften, her body relaxed and warm. Her family was coming in and out although they gave me much privacy during the sessions, just frequently checking in on her. One of her cats came and curled himself up at the nape of her neck, was really drawn to the energy. That same cat jumped into the back of the van before her body was taken and just kind of checked it out. That was really quite sweet.

The last day I was there her daughter was trying to snuggle with her so I created a space on the edge of the bed so that she could sit and lie with her mother and not fall out of bed, just kind of embrace her. Everyone was drawn to her energy even though she was incredibly weak, breathing shallowly but evenly, not able to physically give anyone anything. Every one of her children came to see her, people just gravitated to this circle of energy that was emanating from her. It was soothing, calming, encapsulating, and if it could have spoken it would have said, "All is good, there is nothing to fear." That is what I would say to people about death: there is nothing to fear.

————————————— ••●●●●•• —————————————

I think that the peacefulness that Healing Touch creates is enormous. Because my experiences have only been with people who were ready and open to the next space it made it easier for there to be a sense of peacefulness. My sense is that the Healing Touch smoothed out, softened, created a beautiful energy field. I have seen glitters of silver and gold and blue sparkles everywhere. I don't believe that Healing Touch was totally responsible for it, but it just expanded it in a way.

When we can teach family members some of the techniques it gives them something tangible that they can gift to a loved one who is crossing over, and know that they are doing good, not just for that person but for themselves as well. There are those threads of connection that say, "I'm right here, I'm not turning my back on you, I'm right here." And then again, that power of touch. Healing Touch can be very hands off, but I think there is something very exquisite of the gentle laying on of hands and energy interchange that we feel with the heat and with the touch. There is a level of intimacy of just being present, being profoundly connected, just being with them.

These are the best scenarios, when the person is mentally and emotionally ready to die and the family is supportive, but I know of deaths that have been unpleasant, the person has been agitated and angry and hostile, almost. But it's not so much about the dying process as it is about their living, their life, and what they haven't done, haven't been able to resolve and make sense of. In my private counseling practice I help people finish whatever experiences in their life that they had that were traumatic or unpleasant or confusing to them so they could tidy that up. Then, in the big picture of their life it would allow them to not have to carry that with them when they are in the dying process. So it's a piece of clearing the path.

There is another aspect to death that I became aware of when my dog died. I was always aware of how spiritual she was, she was a therapy dog that went to work with me, just lived by my side, and she touched a lot of people's lives. I held her at the vets as she crossed over, and a week later when I went for my regular appointment with a body worker she said, "You're not in your body, you went over too far with Cloe so I need to call you back." I was aware that something had shifted, that I felt different, but I hadn't realized until then that part of me had gone with Cloe when she left, maybe because I needed to know that she would be okay.

This need to know that our loved one, be it an animal or a human is okay, is such a strong need that I wonder how many people are missing a part of themselves after a death. Does a part of us go with them and we don't even know it, and we need to call it back? In my counseling work with people who have suffered trauma, part of my work is to help them realize that there is a piece that's gone and that they can call it back. For a person who has lost a loved one we can work together to find a way to know that there is still a connection without having to give up a piece of themselves. They can't be together in physical form as before, but the essence of that being, the spiritual piece hasn't gone anywhere; if anything it's strengthened itself.

When I think about how becoming a Healing Touch practitioner has impacted me the simple word is that it has expanded my life, personally and professionally. It has expanded my life with my capacity to love deeply - I probably should say more deeply, I always felt I loved deeply, - it has created a broader space for me to be present without expectation, without anticipation, so that I can merely let life be.

When I do a session I use a general prayer requesting that the work is for one's greater good and that we not be attached to the outcome. I use music if people want it, and I have used some essential oils but it is not a regular part of my practice.

I am struck every time I do a Healing Touch session how palpable the energy is that I sense intuitively, that I feel energetically, that I sense with heat, that I also see, when I use my pendulum, and it does not cease to amaze me how our bodies can heal themselves if we just clear enough of the path so that our body can do its work and blend with the physical body, the emotional body, the spiritual body, the intellectual body in a way that creates a rhythm and a cadence that enhances the existing rhythm and cadence of life that we sometimes are oblivious towards. So expansive: that is interesting to me because I'm not sure I have used that word before when I've thought about it, but I have certainly sensed it.

Massage Therapy Overview

Application

Massage therapy has application for any point in time in a person's life span, from pregnancy, infancy through adulthood, and in the dying process. It induces deep relaxation, helps correct and repair physical imbalances and injuries, helps restore and boost the body's own healing processes, and relieves fear and anxiety. In end-of-life care where recovery is not possible, massage provides physical and emotional comfort from a caring and compassionate presence, and may bring symptom relief where pharmaceuticals alone cannot.

History

Using massage for health and wellbeing has a long history dating back to at least 3,000 BCE in India. Ayurveda, the traditional holistic medical system in India, includes diet and herbalism, aromatherapy, color therapy, sound therapy, and touch therapy. Massage therapy in some form or another is depicted as far back as tomb paintings in Egypt, texts in China dating back to 2700 BCE, practiced by Japanese monks who brought massage techniques from China around 1000 BCE then adapted them into their own system of Shiatsu, in Greece between 800 and 700 BCE, in Rome between 200 and 100 BCE, and in Europe and the United States from the 17th century to the present.

Massage has fallen in and out of favor over the centuries but is currently being widely adopted as a part of accepted health care. Hippocrates advocated massage and exercise for "optimizing body suppleness and tone" and considered it to be "one of the arts with

which a well-rounded physician should be familiar" but requiring lots of hands-on experience in order to be proficient.
http://www.greekmedicine.net/therapies/Massage_and_Bodywork.html

Requirements for licensure or certification

There are no standard requirements for licensure or certification in massage therapy across the United States. Requiring a license in order to practice a profession is set by a state legislature. Proof of competency is required, including graduating from an accredited program with the number of hours of instruction and practice decided upon by the state's legislative body, passing a state exam, and adhering to a set of ethical guidelines.

Certification may be offered by a state, county, city, or other local government agency, and requirements are less stringent than for licensure. Professional certification is a designation sought by a practitioner from a certifying body, not from the government. A massage therapist may choose to become board certified by taking an examination to prove they meet the education, training, and/or experience to show that they have the skills, abilities, knowledge, and attributes to practice as a professional. Board certification is administered by the National Certification Board for Therapeutic Massage and Bodywork (NCBTMB).
http://www.ncbtmb.org

As massage therapy in hospital and hospice settings is becoming more common, the need for specialized training to care for these patients became apparent. The American Hospital Association reports that massage therapy is the number one complementary and alternative integrated medicine service provided in outpatient settings, and the second most popular in inpatient settings.
www.aha.org

Massage schools prepare their graduates to work in private practice and in spas, wellness centers, and sports programs, but not in institutional centers with fragile patients. To rectify this, a 2014 survey asking about the educational requirements, orientation procedures, and competencies of hospital-based massage therapists resulted in the document *Hospital Based Massage Therapy: A Call for Competencies*, which was issued by the Hospital Based Massage Therapy (HBMT) Task Force. https://www.**massage**mag.com/**hospital-based-massage-therapy-call-comp**...

Summary

There are numerous books and articles on the use of massage therapy for overall health and wellbeing, stress relief, pain and anxiety reduction, symptom relief for patients with life-altering illnesses and injuries, and end-of-life care. Massage may bring relief where pharmaceuticals alone cannot, with the added invaluable element of the soothing nature of the work and the calm and compassionate presence of the therapist.

Massage Therapist Interviews

Gayle
Bachelor of Science in Health and Physical Education
Masters in Teaching
Licensed Massage Therapist
Continuing Education Provider in Massage Therapy

Introduction

Gayle is a massage therapist but doesn't do much hands-on herself at this point in her career, having chosen to focus on teaching, supervision, and continuing education for massage therapists. She works at a large teaching hospital.

Interview

I didn't set out to become a massage therapist, it's more like it came and got me. I was a public school teacher and did a year's exchange overseas, and when I got back I came down with a really severe case of chronic fatigue syndrome. I had to quit teaching and go through a long recovery, then an acquaintance said that she was teaching a polarity therapy class before she moved out of the area and that I should take it. It was like a bolt of lightening, I had found what I wanted to do next. I went to massage school, got licensed and was doing some teaching at the school where I graduated when a call came in from the hospital volunteer services coordinator wanting to know if we had students who could come and work with patients. We were asked by the medical board at the hospital to make oncology our home base, so that's how I came to work in my present position. There was no plan on my part, like I said, it just came and got me.

I still work at the same hospital, a large teaching hospital where I oversee the massage therapy program, teach and mentor massage therapists, and do some of the treatments. I'll talk specifically about cancer patients since that is the population that we work with here.

For the most part I teach; I teach massage therapists how to work with people living with cancer, a foundational class, then they can go on and take the chemo infusion class which is a six-day intensive with the inpatients. I work on coordinating the training side and the service side, integrating these. We work with cancer patients who are in treatment: chemo infusion, radiation oncology, and inpatients, providing comfort oriented massage. The massage therapy program started as a clinical training and now has funding for twenty-four hours a week. Sometimes people are in the hospital for end-of-life care but those numbers are very few.

We were volunteer level for about eighteen or nineteen years, which is a long time, so after giving our services for free for so long I have pushed back recently. Massage therapists pay $13,000 to go to massage school, they are licensed by the state, they are not candy stripers. A nurse goes to school longer, although we go to school about the same length of time as an LPN. Nurses are not asked, social workers are not asked to be volunteers. I've said to some of the units who want us to continue to volunteer, "You need to fund this, the only way it's going to be professional and have somebody show up every week for their shift, time after time, is to pay them." The hospital wants our services but they don't want to pay, they don't see the value until they actually pony up some money and go, "Wow, it's good having somebody show up on a regular basis." Then the staff starts relating to the therapist much differently.

I've had some success, we got funding through a corporation grant for twenty-four hours a week in oncology, which shifted things immeasurably. There is somebody on cardiology for a four-hour shift and somebody at the children's hospital working with parents. Nurses are now beginning to ask us if there is anything that we can do to help alleviate the discomfort from specific conditions, such as from swelling, rather than just seeing us as providing comfort care.

Massage is getting funded at some hospitals, but a need that is just beginning to get attention is the specialized training that a massage therapist needs to have in order to work with hospital patients. A shortcoming of our work is that there isn't a protocol in place to take students through their studies, followed by a practicum with supervision and assessment.

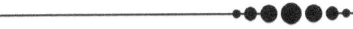

I'll give you an overview of the work that we do. In the outpatient hematology clinic we see a lot of bone marrow patients being prepped for bone marrow transplants, induction chemo. These are patients that are seen for several years, so they may come in at any point in their treatment. Other patients are being treated for leukemia or lymphoma and they are in and out for chemo and fluids and transfusions.

When a massage therapist goes into the outpatient infusion clinic the nurses are now attuned enough to us and what we do that they will suggest that we start with a particular patient. The patients are in lounge-type chairs with a footrest that kicks up, so we do a foot massage and if possible some massage around the shoulders and neck. However, some of the clinics are so crowded that there isn't enough space to do anything except at the feet.

The typical foot massage lasts for twenty minutes, and because of the way the room is laid out everybody can see what's happening. If someone is watching, just looking, you can catch their eye, wheel on over to stand at their side and introduce yourself, and talk about the massage service. People change their chemo day so they can be there when there is a massage therapist. They tell us that they experience less pain and anxiety and feel relaxed. We've had times when the nurses are having trouble getting the line in, so they will do a hot pack where they want the line to go, the massage therapist will do a foot massage, and bingo, that relaxation helps the vein pop so they can get the line in. That's always pretty dramatic.

Our inpatient care covers two floors, which is a lot of pancreatic, gynecological, blood/brain barrier disruptions, ovarian, colorectal, neck and throat patients. These patients are in and out in a week or weeks, whereas bone marrow transplant patients can be in for months, and after that they can be in and out because they can be in and out of crisis. A lot of the patients on the medical oncology floor suffer from swelling. It's a combination of ascites, an accumulation of fluid in the peritoneal cavity causing abdominal swelling; albumin levels off which throws off the fluid balance in the body; and interstitial swelling, the accumulation of fluids between the cells, so it's just an overall condition which probably makes them as uncomfortable as anything.

Here's a classic tale. We worked with a patient in the process of having white blood cells collected for the stem cell transplant, but she had chemo induced peripheral neuropathy from the chemo she had had prior to starting the bone marrow transplant. It was really bad, so bad that they gave her morphine for it, which is kind of an unusual thing to give for peripheral neuropathy. It didn't work, but five minutes of massage did work, that was the only thing that worked. It didn't relieve it permanently, but it gave her a break from the pain.

We had another patient who had a bone marrow transplant who was suffering from a lot of neck pain. They were trying a lot of different things with him from morphine to hot packs but nothing was really doing it. They asked me to work with him, it had to do with his catheter, the way it was placed, and the massage helped him more than morphine.

Typically a person does not want as robust massage as prior to their cancer treatment. There are side effects to adjust for, there's just something about cancer treatment that leaves a footprint on a person. As they go into recovery and get stronger the massage can be a little bit more effortful, they can have more robust massages, but even then they do not want as much as prior to their treatment. The touch is lighter, they can have holds, anybody can have anything pretty much all through the process, it's just knowing how to adjust to what is going on with their treatments and their bodies and what they want.

Let's say you are a shiatsu practitioner, which is a firmer pressure on the points, but for the person in treatment is very gentle, just barely resting on a point with minimal pressure. Maybe the session needs to be shorter, less information given to the body because there is already so much input given to them with medications and drugs and insurance. Then as people move into recovery and they are working to rejuvenate their body they can have a more restorative session. I like the word restorative because it's a goal of returning a person to as much full function as possible.

I don't often work with patients at end of life although recently I worked with a man who was probably on his last night of life. During the day prior to his discharge from the hospital to go home and enter hospice I did a foot massage with him. I put lotion on his feet and worked and worked with him for an hour. I wouldn't normally do an hour session, but I just stayed at his feet and kept talking, and it was him just talking about his children, about his life, reviewing his life, and he blessed me.

Before long he was readmitted to the hospital for end-of-life care, I suppose because he needed complex care that they couldn't give him at home through hospice. The last night that I worked with him he wasn't cognizant very much but he knew I was there. The family was sitting vigil in the room, and they were so grateful for the care that I was giving him. They needed a break, the nurses were in and out, so they were really grateful that somebody was going to be there with him.

I am comfortable with death and I understand that things have natural life spans, including human beings, projects, there are all kinds of ways that things come to an end. I think it's having your pulse on that time of when; when is it time? For those people who believe in an afterlife it doesn't seem so horrible that somebody has moved on; it's not that they are completely gone, it's just that they've transitioned.

Letting go into death can be difficult sometimes. It can be the patient who wants more treatments, or the family who doesn't want to give up on their loved one, or the doctor who wants to do as the family requests even when he or she knows that there is no hope. We had the situation in my family when it was time for my dad to let go. He had had an aortic valve replacement, which was a bit of a rocky thing, but then his small intestine died. I don't know if they ever knew why, but he was going to have to be on a feeding tube and my mom said, "There's no way he is going to want to do that, no way." So they let things take their natural course, but my youngest brother couldn't cope with that at all. So we got fifteen people together, the gastroenterologist, the heart surgeon, the social worker, all these people together to say to him, "There's nothing else we can do." He had to hear it from this whole room full of people.

I think the nurses are the ones who are connected to the patient the most deeply, and they are the midwives into this process; they're the ones who have to open this space for the family, for everybody, including the physicians. This is me spouting off, but it's just sort of a feeling I have that the nurses have to hold the space for the physicians and for the family, so they are a midwife to the dying. It's because nursing is a feminine thing, and I think death, there's something feminine, it's part of the feminine. The masculine is much more about the sparking, adventure, out there, but nursing is a feminine thing, it's about holding, it's circular.

The nurses were really helpful when my dad was dying. They were the ones that you'd ask, "What would you do if it was your dad?" The doctors weren't there, they do their rounds, "Here we are, we're here for five minutes, how's your pain?" And they enter something on the computer. "How's your bowels?" And they enter that into the computer. That's what I've noticed, because I'm in the room sometimes when they round, but it's the nurse that's there holding the process; they're holding the process for the family and they're holding the process for the patient.

The nurses were the most helpful to me, personally. There was one nurse who had lost her dad maybe six weeks before and she just ponied up and admitted it, didn't pretend, have the professional façade, which was helpful to know that she was just a little bit ahead of me. And then the other nurse, when we were trying to decide to extubate my dad because he just kept going and going, he needed to die but he just kept going and going, and I said, "What would you do if it was your dad?" She said, "I'd take the tube out." It's that honest, totally honest, human-to-human relationship that was the most helpful.

Massage therapy is also a human-to-human relationship that provides many benefits that we don't often think about. It creates a space for people to talk about the things that are important to them, like their families, and the time for life review. It helps bring order out of chaos; there's something about touch that helps bring a sense of order and calmness. When a person gets a diagnosis of cancer, let's say, but it could be any type of serious illness, the limbic system goes bonkers and you can hardly think. That happens all along the way, and when in the hospital it is traumatizing for people and there is a lot of chaos, it's really hard to settle down. With the benefit of massage they are able to make decisions more easily, decisions come faster and they have more clarity. When you can calm the limbic system it will naturally have some effect on a person's levels of pain and anxiety.

Because I was so sick for so long I came to believe that illness polishes the soul and it's hard, but lots of things polish the soul. Not everyone will feel this way, but during my illness I felt that the huge changes occurring in my life were somehow for the best. I think we suffer when we feel hopeless. I certainly felt hopeless at times but I was fortunate that there were some things that helped sustain me. I had four months of paid sick leave from my teaching job and then I was able to get disability. I had enough to get by so I could just relax into it, and a lot of people don't have that.

But once you've lost your ability to work and have an income it makes its imprint on you, it creates an insecurity about money. It's easy for me to put myself into a cancer patient's shoes, or anybody with serious medical problems, because of my experience. The anxiety about how to pay for one's medical care is, I believe, an underlying fear that as Americans we carry. It does make me wonder about the relationship between money, either peace of mind about it or anxiety over it, and one's ability to recover from illness. In the United Kingdom a person would not have to worry about losing their house in order to pay for medical care.

During my illness and recovery I learned to do a lot of self-care. I had to pay out of pocket for everything because there is no mainstream treatment for what I had. I did a lot of nutritional supplements, cleanses, and a healthy diet. I walk my dog and have a weekly massage. Another part of my self-care is I don't put myself in environments that sap my energy. I do the kind of work that I do because it supports me, it supports my cells, it's quiet, it's peaceful. I don't hang out with people and in environments that don't feel good to me. Sometimes I think that's a shortcoming on my part, like I should be able to handle it, but when you understand energy you understand how it affects you, both positively and negatively. Part of self-care is to be with people who nurture us rather than drain us.

Working with patients does not drain me, it's not a difficult part of my work. What is difficult is the politics and the professional isolation. Since massage therapy is still rarely a paid position there is usually only one therapist on duty at a time for only a few hours each week so there is not the peer support and debriefing that many other professions have. I want us to be able to grow into a respected profession in which our work is valued. It used to be that nurses cleaned the rooms, they did the physical therapy and occupational therapy, they did simple massage like back rubs, and now we have all these separate disciplines that I would describe as having grown into themselves but massage therapy has lagged behind.

In order for that to happen I think it will take a combination of us respecting ourselves as professionals, specialized training to work with patients, requests for our work from patients and other staff who see the benefits to patients and families, evidence based outcomes, grants from foundations, and money budgeted for paid positions. There is already a great deal of research on the benefits of massage; pain and anxiety reduction has been studied extensively, for example, so I'm not sure what we need to do next to be granted full-fledged professional status with commensurate pay. That's the frustration, the politics of it all.

Mary
Registered Nurse
Holistic Nurse-Board Certified
Licensed Massage Therapist
Therapeutic Touch Practitioner

Introduction

Mary is an RN and a licensed massage therapist who has a private practice. She is frequently invited to train staff and work with patients, most recently for hospice and in assisted living centers. She was able to bring a perspective to the field of nursing and massage that younger professionals are not due to the fact that protocols have changed over the years. Much of the interview highlights the simple act of touch and light massage to a person's wellbeing.

Interview

I grew up in a small logging community in the Pacific Northwest where most women never moved on, they married a logger, settled down, and raised a family. I never wanted to do that, so out of the three of us girls in the family I was the first one to go to college over my stepfather's objections. He didn't think a girl should go to college because it was just a waste of time since she would end up getting married anyway and never use the education.

My mother supported me in my desire for an education, and because of my grades I was able to get scholarships and I ended up going to the School of Nursing at the University of Puget Sound. I was in the program for four years, the first year attending the college and the other three years living in the nursing dorm and basically working for the hospital to get the nursing education. We got fantastic experience doing that, and then we went to Vancouver, BC for our pediatrics rotations, then to Seattle for our tuberculosis rotation, then to Steilacoom for our mental health rotation. We had really, really good hands-on training. These three-year diploma nurses are highly regarded as the best trained hands-on nurses that there are.

In the fundamentals of nursing one of the basic things we learned with a bed bath that RNs did was a 15 minute back rub. Every patient got a back rub in the evening before bed; it was called pm care. That's just what you did; it wasn't an LPN, it wasn't a nurse's aid, you didn't even have them then, the RNs did them. You're the ones who had the load, you're the ones who had to take care of the patients you had, and you were responsible for them.

The 15 minute back rub, but it's not 15 minutes any more, same back rub, it's 3-5 minutes. When I ask nursing students "Do you know that this is in the fundamentals book?" and they look at me with like, "What?" So I say, "When you go back to your room look it up; it's right there." And they're blown away. And I ask, "Are you taught anything about touch?" "No, just how to handle people with procedural touch, how to be safe, but not comfort touch, not comfort."

I was really attracted to that for some reason, the touch piece of it, and saw what happened with sleeping better, reducing medications, decreased stress, emotional needs, I mean, you actually have this time when you get to know a patient during this 15 minutes. After nursing school my main job was in an allergy clinic, but I never lost my interest in using touch as part of a patient's health care. I taught child birth education classes for about three years, and it was during this time that I was introduced to Therapeutic Touch. It opened up all kinds of things for me including using crystals as part of an energy healing session. There was no certification process when I took the training so I just played with friends and relatives, asking if I could experiment with using crystals, and asking them if they noticed any difference when I did. They always had a different reaction whenever I used them; the healing modality seemed to get stronger and more effective. It was interesting.

I initially learned about Therapeutic Touch when I attended a lecture by the famous healer Olga Worrall (1906-1985). She showed a movie clip of some of the things she did, and she showed a movie clip with Dolores Krieger doing Therapeutic Touch. I had never heard of anything like that, never seen anything like that, and I thought, "I want to know more about that." She also showed some movies of things she did at Harvard where there were a lot of experiments done with her to study the healing process.

Some time after this lecture I got a flyer in the mail about a workshop on healing with all the great healing people from all the great religions, and Dolores Krieger was on the program. I didn't pay a whole lot of attention to it, but then it came to me two other times from other people so I got it three times and I thought, "Okay, I think I'm supposed to pay attention to this."

It was a three or four day conference and one of the most outstanding conferences I have ever gone to. There were hundreds of people there and leaders from all the great religions and traditions: Buddhist, Hindu, Islam, Jewish, Christianity, Native American, and more, all these healing-type people from all over the world; I can still see it to this day. At one point in the conference they were all sitting up on the stage together in a semi-circle and the moderator asked them: "What do you think you all have in common?" The thing that every single person said was love; we are here to love one another. We say it in different ways but that's the path, love.

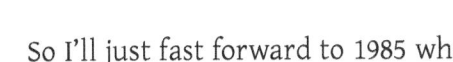

So I'll just fast forward to 1985 when I got my massage license. I had this great vision that I'd be able to bring touch into nursing more if I had my massage license, but I was wrong. I didn't really get in the door with nursing until 2002 when I got in on the ground floor to help develop an integrative medicine clinic in the cancer department at one of the local hospitals. We got a one-year grant from the Susan G. Komen Foundation to teach diet and exercise to breast cancer patients: that was the biggest step into integrative medicine that the hospital could take at that time. Later they added a naturopath, then they added a massage therapist, then two more naturopaths/acupuncturists, and we ended up with five therapists.

I was the assistant to the doctor who was creating the program and since it was only a three-day-a week job it gave me time to make a lot of contacts with the nurses in the hospital. I was trying to promote the importance of touch, trying to see if we could get it in somewhere, and thinking through what I would teach if I could do a class for nurses. I knew that if I said, "I want to teach your nurses how to do a 15 minute back rub on a patient on the evening shift," they would shut the door in my face. They would say, "You're absolutely out of touch, you crazy lady." I knew I couldn't approach it that way so I just kept asking myself what I could do to get touch in the door in a way that would be accepted.

I finally got the attention of the nurse in charge of nursing education and the nurse-educators under her. They said, "Alright, we want our staff, all sixty of them, to be trained in the importance of touch. We want you to teach the supervisors first and then teach the rest of our staff." A nurse who was working on his PhD at the time became my assistant in putting everything together. It was wonderful. He pulled research, we decided what would be taught in the class, we created a notebook, and the program became known as *Re-Awakening Touch as Patient Care: The Red Bear Training.* Red Bear is a red teddy bear that is the mascot of all the workshops that I do now. Everybody who takes one of my classes gets a little photo of Red Bear with these instructions: "When you look at him ask two questions. The first question is 'Who needs touch in my life today? Who do I need to reach out to, who do I need to make a phone call to, who do I need to write a note to, who do I need to give a hug to, who do I need to say hello to, who needs touch, any form of touch today?' The other question is, 'What do I need to do to take care of myself? Do I need a rest? Do I need to listen to music? Do I need to do some meditation, take a walk, get a massage? What do I need to do to keep me going?' " That's Red Bear. There are now about 3,000 of them out there. I tell people that with time they will probably forget me, but they will never forget Red Bear and what that represents for them.

Since I only had an hour for the workshop, I decided that I would teach three techniques of simple comfort touch in two-minute exercises. I wanted them to learn what they could do, and the difference you can make in a patient's experience in the hospital if you only have two minutes, even one minute, but the only way you are going to know that is if you experience it as a giver and as a receiver.

We start out working in pairs and one person is #1, the other #2. The first thing I always say in the class is, "When you meet somebody for the first time, what do we usually do?" We usually shake hands. So I say, "Person #1, I want you to take your partner's hand and just shake hands." Then they switch, with #2, extending their hand first and shaking hands with their partner. Then I have them do it again, but this time I instruct them to place their other hand over the top of their partner's hand. It doesn't have to linger there very long, just a brief hold, and then I ask them to share what that was like. They will say, "Well, that was different," and I ask, "What was different about it?" They say things like, "It was more connected, it was more personal, it was more caring."

So here's the point, I say. If I do this, I come into your room as the nurse, I come in and shake your hand in the typical fashion and I can just keep going, but if I come in and do the hand over the hand handshake I have to make a connection, whether it's for two seconds, one second, you cannot look away and do a two-handed handshake. So this is what I always teach in the very beginning. If they don't go away with anything else I encourage them to do the two-handed handshake. I tell them they don't have to hang out there and be uncomfortable, just touch. Do it wherever you are where you would typically be shaking hands and see how people respond: they will know there is that caring piece in it.

The second thing we do is a hand rub. I don't use the word massage because the elderly, for the most part, are not familiar with where the world of massage has gone, and if you come in and ask, "May I massage your hand, or massage your back," or whatever, you are going to get a push back because they are thinking of it in different terms, like the massage parlors of ill repute rather than therapeutic massage.

So we're going to say a hand rub, or "May I put some lotion on your hands because it helps you relax or sleep better or take a rest; is that okay?" It's better than saying, "Can I massage your hand?" Massage can be hard, it can be painful, and I'll say to the nurses in the class, "I don't want any of you to even think about being a massage therapist, that's not what this touch is about, this touch is about comfort. So you're to take the patient's hand and you are to rub slowly and all over with lotion that you have warmed, doing each individual finger. In the class I tell them the important thing here is to do the hand rub as slowly as you can, and the next hardest thing is you cannot talk. So you cannot talk for four minutes, two minutes each hand, not talking. The reason is that I want you to see what it's like to fully experience being a giver and being a receiver, and you cannot do that if you're talking, you're distracting yourself.

Both of these things are very interesting, the not talking and the slowing down. People want to go faster, so I watch the class and I will say, "Some of you still need to slow down. If you slow down that two minutes is going to seem like a really long time, but if you're going fast your partner (or your patient) is going to wish you were done and just get the heck out of there, it's not going to be relaxing. As they are doing this exercise I count down in thirty second intervals so they know where they are in the process, and I also say, "Be aware of where your mind is. If you're thinking about where you need to be next when you get out of here, going home, cooking dinner, or something you didn't do, bring that mind back to this hand." I remind them that if they are thinking about something else the patient will know that they're not there, they will feel it in their touch, so come back, be present.

The next thing I have them do is to do the same exercise but with gloves on. The giver will wear the same kind of exam gloves that the nurse and aides wear to change dressings and all the other things they do in the hospital. They are taught that gloves protect them from infections and protects the patient as well, so it serves as a barrier between the caregiver and the patient. What I want to show them in class is that you can still do meaningful, warm, caring touch even if you have your gloves on if your mind and your heart is in the place to send the energy. It doesn't matter that there is a glove on, it doesn't matter that there is a foot of blankets or anything else, it's your intention and what you're bringing to that person.

Everybody is skeptical – gloves? I say, "Just trust, we're not going to talk about it until it's over because I don't want to put anything into your mind." So they put the gloves on, they put the lotion on the gloves, and they do the hand rub on their partner. In some classes people will respond to the experience on both ends of the spectrum to "I hated that, I didn't feel like I was even close, I like the skin contact," but others will say, "I couldn't tell any difference, particularly when I was the one getting it." These different reactions give us a chance to talk about what happened, and mostly what happened is the attitude about wearing the gloves. If you do the procedure with the attitude of resistance toward wearing the gloves that will be sensed by the patient, whereas if you are fine with it and just have the attitude that you are going to do something nice for the patient, that feeling will also be transmitted. So it's not the gloves that make a difference, it's the person wearing the gloves. I used to do massage in a class for cancer and stem cell transplant patients and we always wore gloves. They couldn't tell because we always came with the caring and loving component.

The last thing we do in class is have one of the partners sit in a chair, the other person stands behind them and puts their hands on their partner's shoulders, holds for about thirty seconds, then brushes out and away along the shoulders for about thirty seconds, then hold the outsides of the shoulders for thirty seconds, then a little more brushing, then holding the shoulders close to the neck, then a deep breath and both giver and receiver relax, then trade places. After this I tell some stories, beginning with the one that got me thinking about teaching touch.

I was working for a rheumatologist and patients would come in with redness, swelling at the wrists and other joints, so if you were the patient and you came in and you showed me your hand I would just intuitively pick up the hand and the wrist and hold it. One day a patient said, "That feels so good." It was instantaneous, that's all I did, and I'm thinking, "What happened here that would get that response that fast?" So now I teach that minimal touch can get a full body response by doing even just one hand. If you don't have time for a hand rub you can get the same kind of response by just holding the hand, and if you can do the sandwich, one hand on top and the other underneath, even more healing energy will be generated. It doesn't always have to be the hand, though; touching any part of the body will create that healing response. We also talk about how we communicate with patients when they have to do something that hurts them, letting them know that we understand and will be as gentle as possible. The same procedures can be done in a brisk and businesslike manner, or in a slower and more caring manner with that human connection. It takes only a few moments to make that connection but it makes a great deal of difference to the patient.

One day I was taking a class on massage for cancer patients when I was asked to go to the ICU. I went up and here's this young man, probably in his early 20s, lying on the bed with every imaginable hook-up, on a ventilator, and either in a coma or unconscious. His dad was in the room, just kind of pacing, and I asked him if it was alright if I touched his son. The only place I could see to touch him was on his shoulder, and I'm wondering what I could possibly do, so I said that I would ask the nurse and see if it is okay to touch him there. The nurse came in and said that it was okay, and I demonstrated the very light touch that I would be doing and she said that was fine.

I washed my hands and I went over to the young man and introduced myself because I knew at some level he would know I was there, maybe could even hear me, who I was, and that I was going to do some relaxation massage up here on his shoulder to see if that would bring him some relief. So I started rubbing ever so slightly, and when I first touched him he took this big breath and I thought, "Okay, we've connected." And then his monitor changed, his respirations went down, his blood pressure lowered, and I'm watching it all happening right there in front of me. After a few minutes the nurse runs in and says, "What are you doing? Whatever you're doing, keep doing it, it's doing all the right things." I never talked to him, just did the gentle massage. I don't know what ultimately happened with him.

In the rheumatology clinic I worked in I had a mother and a young lady come in who was dying from a connective tissue disease. The young woman was crying, in a lot of pain, and the mother was distraught. So I said, "If you like I could just do a light back rub for her right now and see if it will help her pain." She said, "That would be wonderful." So I did the traditional massage from nursing, not what I learned in massage school, a slow stroke massage up the center of the back, across the shoulders, down, around the hips. The pain decreased and she stopped crying. When I was done the mother said, "Why hasn't anybody taught me this?" I told her I couldn't answer that but I could teach her how to do it. Before long the doctor came in and I was a bit concerned about what the mother was going to tell him since he didn't believe in any sort of complementary and alternative medicine, but when he came out of the room he said, "Call the hospital and arrange for her to have a massage twice a day for every day that she's in the hospital." I said okay, and nothing else was ever said.

My whole message is comfort and caring, helping people to sleep, require less medication, reduce pain and anxiety, just to be there for them. I tell nurses to engage the family in comfort care for their loved one. Often family members don't know what to do and can sometimes be sitting in the room but completely ignoring the person in the bed and the nurse can go over, or I can go over and say, "Can I teach you something to do when I'm not here? Let me show you." Let's just say it is a mother and son, and I go to the son and take his hand and say, "If you go sit by your mom and you just hold her hand like this so she knows you're there for her, I know it will really help." You can't just tell the person "When I leave, will you please go over there and hold your mother's hand, I know it will really help her." You can't do that because he may never have held his mother's hand and he may not know how to, so you show him what it feels like, that level of touch. So I try to do that, empower people.

One of the quotes I give to people in my classes is from Florence Nightingale. "What nursing has to do . . . is to put the patient in the best condition for nature to act upon him." She used touch and massage and knew that if you can get the body in a comfort state it can access its ability to heal, but if it's in a stress state it can't. It shuts down the immune system and everything else you need to get well. So whatever you use to put the body into the parasympathetic mode rather than the sympathetic you are on the road to healing.

Stress activates the sympathetic nervous system, which raises blood pressure, among other things. One day I had an 85-year-old woman come who was suffering from severe high blood pressure. I asked her if she would like me to rub her neck and shoulders a little bit before the doctor came in and she said, "Oh, that would be so wonderful. I did that for my husband before he died, he was sick for a very long time and I massaged him every day but no one has ever touched me." So we did some touch and after I was done, maybe five minutes, I asked her if she minded if I took her blood pressure again. It had dropped 30 points. That poor woman, she was just hurting so much. I tell this story in my classes to bring awareness of the elderly who, in most cases, will not ask for touch but they are lying there waiting for you to reach out.

One day I was doing some massage with cancer patients and taking some photos for a massage therapy book when we got word that there was a lady who had come in for her chemotherapy but they wanted to postpone it because her blood pressure was too high. Her son had driven her in from her home 75 miles away and having to go back home just seemed crazy. So I went over to her and asked, "Would you like to try some massage? Maybe, just maybe it would lower your blood pressure and you could stay and you wouldn't have to go back home." I did a back massage, neck and shoulders, and it dropped enough that she was able to stay and receive her chemotherapy treatment. I could see that her son was obviously stressed, so I said, "Come on, let's give you a backrub." He finally agreed and was grateful for it.

There are just an endless number of stories about the power of touch. There was a patient on a gurney in the hospital hallway, waiting to be wheeled into the operating room, when a nun who was passing through the hall paused by the gurney, took his hand and she said, "I'll pray for you." He was so touched by her kindness that after his recovery he wanted to give something in return so he donated several of his paintings, which hang in the hospital's main lobby, all because someone reached out and touched him.

It can be so simple. I had a hospice patient whose daughter wanted massage and touch for their mother. I went to the home and the mother said she would like some touch, so I did some very light touch on her back and face, and just held her face for a few moments. After I was done I asked the family who were gathered around watching what was happening if they would like me to show them what I was doing.

They were not a very touchy family but everybody said yes, they were interested, so I gave each of them some touch. I gave the son a shoulder massage and said, "You can do this for your mom, this is the pressure that you use." I asked the daughter if I could show her what she could do for her mom just in terms of holding her face. The next time I went to the home the daughter said, "I want you to know that I went up and I held my mom's face like this, really soft, and she just loved it." That was a sweet story.

When I was at the workshop with Olga Worrall she said to me, "I am going to tell you a couple of things that I never want you to forget," and believe me, I haven't. I had mentioned that I would argue with the doctor because he didn't believe in what I did and she said, "Don't ever argue with your doctor again, it serves no good," and I never did. The other thing she said is "Healing energy knows exactly where to go and what to do; all you have to do is call it forth. So whenever you are doing something for your patient, whether it's taking blood pressure or anything, just call forth in your mind and your heart healing energy to do whatever it needs to do. You don't have to say diddly-squat or do anything, call it forth within you. You see somebody in the elevator, call forth healing energy, wherever you are call forth the healing energy. Just know that it's always there and it knows exactly what to do."

Acupuncture Overview

Application

Interest in Eastern medicine waxes and wanes, even in the East, with Western medicine in the United States currently in a period in which there is increased interest which is leading to more research.

Acupuncture is based on the theory that there are meridians, or "energy highways," or "energy channels" within the body along which energy travels, referred tas chi or vital life force. The energy flow along the meridians nourish all parts of the body and if something impedes or blocks the flow it affects a person's health.

Much of the reluctance of Western Medicine to accept acupuncture is that the meridians are not physical structures like arteries, blood vessels, and nerves, and therefore cannot be proven to exist through standard medical means. In addition, there is no agreement on how and why it works, although the research does show that it works for many health conditions with no negative side effects.

Treatment consists of very fine needles inserted at an acupuncture point or points along the meridian or meridians to correspond to the condition being treated. The depth of insertion is shallow, often only ¼" to ½" and described by most recipients as painless. The type of acupuncture used by the practitioner, the condition being treated, the status of the patient, and other factors will determine the length of time for any one treatment and the course of treatment over time.

Research cited in the article "Palliative Care," by the British Acupuncture Council www.acupuncture.org.uk discusses the use of acupuncture for the following conditions in palliative and end-of-life care.

Pain	Fatigue
Dry mouth	Lymphedema
Nausea and vomiting	Insomnia
Breathlessness	Depression
Hot flushes	Gastrointestinal upsets

History

As with most if not all ancient medical practices it is impossible to firmly state a date when acupuncture became a part of patient care. It was described in The Yellow Emperor's Classic of Internal Medicine dating from about 100 BCE, and was officially recognized as an independent specialty by the Imperial Medical Bureau of the Tang Government, founded in 618.

Early in the 20th Century, proposals were passed by the Chinese government with the intent to ban all forms of traditional Chinese medicine in favor of Western medicine. In 1950 the official policy changed to encourage the study of traditional Chinese medicine and to integrate the two approaches, East and West, to offset the weaknesses of each and offer the best of integrative medicine to patients.

Requirements for licensure and certification

There is no national standard for licensing and certification, with each state setting its own requirements. Conditions for licensing are graduating from an accredited school and passing the National Certification Commission for Acupuncture and Oriental Medicine (NCCAOM) examination. Accredited schools have rigorous academic and experiential requirements. The website www.thebestschools.org under the article titled "The 20 Best Acupuncture Schools in the US" gives a thorough overview of requirements for graduation from their programs.

Kathryn F. Weymouth, PhD

Summary

The research on acupuncture for many different issues is ongoing, and is showing great promise in some, as in pain management, and less or unknown in others. The website for the National Center for Complementary and Integrative Health, www.nccih.nih.gov, publishes research findings, and among those findings is the safety and lack of side effects from acupuncture treatments. As consumers are becoming more interested in receiving health care that has fewer negative side effects, acupuncture has a place in integrative medicine.

Acupuncturist Interview

Gwen
Bachelor of Arts in Physical Anthropology
Licensed Acupuncturist
Certified Chinese Herbalist
Clinical Supervisor at the National College of
Naturopathic Medicine, Portland, Oregon
Owner, Acupuncture Clinic

Introduction

Gwen has a degree in anthropology and studied Native American medicine and Western herbs, then developed an interest in the Asian approach to acupuncture and herbs. In 1989 she enrolled in the National College of Naturopathic Medicine where she was a student for three years, as well as graduating from the Oregon College of Oriental Medicine. She currently is a clinical supervisor at the naturopathic college and is in private practice as a licensed acupuncturist.

Interview

While I was still a student at the naturopathic college I took a trip to Sri Lanka for a summer and spent three months in a hospital where I was doing acupuncture six days a week, treating twelve people a day. Before I left the United States I had never put a needle into anybody, so it quickly threw me into what it was like to treat people with acupuncture. It was very intense and I learned so much. I was twenty-five at that time and I thought, "I really want to do this and I don't want to do the naturopathic program anymore." I had finished three years and only had a year left, but the conviction of wanting to do more with the acupuncture was so strong that when I returned home I dropped out of naturopathic school. I loved the subtlety of the acupuncture, how it seemed to have such a profound healing in a kind of deeper energetic sense than the actual more kind of gross herbs in physical medicine.

After dropping out I focused completely on acupuncture and Chinese herbs. It was a big transition for me. My grandfather had been a surgeon, it felt like there was a lot of pride, my name, I was going to be a doctor, and now I was just going to be the acupuncturist. But there was actually something freeing about that, as well.

Then I moved and got more immersed in a Japanese style of acupuncture. In a very general sense, Chinese acupuncture can be a little more intense, more physical, usually more palpable, and in Japanese there's a little more subtlety with it, so I was drawn to that. The needles are much finer, they're barely in the skin, it's not about getting anybody to feel anything, it's more about trusting what's already happening in the body and working with that, working with that inherent wisdom more than setting an agenda.

When I graduated in 1994 I was offered a job at a ten-bed hospice house for AIDS patients. At that time someone would be admitted and within two or three weeks they were actively dying. So really quick, and the death from AIDS then was so drastic, so horrible, it was a horrible death. I felt in a way that I was thrown into the deep end: I loved the work but I had no idea what I was doing. As soon as I walked in the door I remember the smell and the feeling of just not knowing what to do. But I loved the intensity of it, I loved how real it was. People weren't talking about the weather, there was no pretense, it was all just "This is the process and I'm dying and I'm going to talk to you about what's really going on."

So I loved that and at the same time I felt ill-equipped. But it was a training, and what it did, it helped me to rely on things like the pulse system, touch people and feel where they were at in that moment. I would meet someone one week and a few days later they would be actively dying and wouldn't be able to communicate with me, so I would rely more on taking their pulse to know what was happening. It was this on-the-job training that allowed me to develop the fine-tuned feedback that I still use to this day, learning how to know where to start, what to do, if it's too much or too little, if it's helping or not helping. Not only that, but when I didn't know what to do I would go inside and ask, so my internal sense, my internal guidance of what to do was also honed. Of course the training that I had had was completely sufficient, it was just the lack of experience on my part, and having people be so sick and not having much communication, not much feedback. So providing hospice care was a doorway into developing these skills, in a sense a doorway into myself.

When I work with a patient I start with the pulse to find out what is showing up and what needs the most attention. The training that I've had was with a doctor on the East coast, there were probably fifteen of us whom he's trained, and this is a very elaborate, very thorough system of using the pulse to determine what is going on in a patient's body. When I have a new patient they have forty-five minutes where they sit there, it's not even an intake, it's just me taking their pulse; it's a lot of time and a lot of attention. It's strange for some people, but most of the time it feels absolutely kind and lovely to be listened to in such depth. I have a woman with pancreatic cancer right now and she's in a lot of pain, but when I take her pulse she just starts to relax and she says it feels like I am so deeply listening to her and it brings her so much joy. I think it's part of being seen, being heard, in such a deep way that there is some healing that happens; it feels like there's a communication, a connection formed between us, starting with the pulse. For some people this is the first time that level of contact and communication has happened, and yes, that aspect of being seen. When I work with students at the naturopathic college I am always asking them, "Where are you? When you're with a patient and if you're running around thinking about eighteen things, what this person might need, what the next person might need, that's all getting in the way of your presence, your ability to pick up the pulse, your ability to really be there as you are touching them."

In the system I've been trained in, you're trained to feel what's really going well, what's really stable, and what's breaking down and where there is even a hint of instability. Cancers, mental illness, autoimmune diseases, these are all secondary to a system that's breaking down; they don't just come out of nowhere. When the system starts to break down, to lose integrity, it starts to show symptoms. Sometimes symptoms are missed, but it certainly is evident in somebody's pulse. Maybe the rate will increase or change, maybe the rhythm will change, or it will just be a feeling. You can feel in the pulse certain qualities emerge, like slippery or pounding. When they're pounding and then they're dropping to an absent or a feeble, and they're back to pounding, this is a picture of chaos. Trying to feel into how much chaos, and being that this is in essence a very preventative medicine, we are trying to get some of that before you actually have manifestation of an illness. Energetically it should show up first in the pulse, it could be five years down the road before that chaos manifests into the illness. You can feel when someone is about to get a cold, you can feel it three days away, so hopefully you can give them what they need and hope the cold will not completely finish the cycle and turn into a cold. So it's the same thing with something about to emerge in a few days' time, a chronic disease, or a serious illness; you can kind of see it coming.

Acupuncture as a medical specialty is gaining much more acceptance than when I first started. It used to be met with comments like, "You could be spreading hepatitis around with those needles," and just the general attitude dismissing anything out of the Western model of mainstream medicine. When I was treating people at the hospice house and at nursing homes back in the 80s and early 90s the doctors wouldn't really look at me, or they would pretend they didn't know what I was doing. Not that long ago I had a patient in intensive care with a stroke and the doctors essentially said that I shouldn't be there, so I quickly did the treatment and left. Now some hospitals have acupuncturists on staff, and even if a doctor is not all that familiar with it, hearing the beneficial results from his patients is making a difference. I remember when I first worked at the hospice house none of the patients were very open to receiving acupuncture but I would treat the staff and when they could say, "I just got acupuncture for my headache and now its gone," it created more openness to it.

To show how things are changing, I got a call asking if I would be available to go to the hospital. "This family needs help; their daughter is dying of colon cancer and she can't breathe." So I went over right away.

The woman is thirty years old, dying of colon cancer, and she was having a portal backup. So basically she was completely jaundiced and swelling and couldn't breathe, and of course there was all this anxiety and panic over her not being able to breathe, just kind of suffocating. This was one of those situations where the room was full of people, family and doctors, and they are all saying, "Oh, we're so glad you're here." I checked the point on her wrist that opens up the chest, there are probably ten points that do very specific things and they do them so well, and this one opens up the chest. So I did that point and a couple of others and she started to be able to breathe, it was a dramatic difference. Her parents called me later and asked if I could please come every day, so I went daily until she died.

In my work at the hospice house I started to see the differences in how people die. There are those who go with a great deal of acceptance, some with less, some with none. This young woman was one of the people who so inspired me, she was so filled with grace, as was the whole experience. I would be there everyday for my hour, just there, just trying to sit there and hang out with her pulse, and she would have people come in and she would say goodbye to them. On the last day, the day she died, I was there, it was in the morning, she brought her parents in and she said, "You've given me this, and you've given me that, you've always done this for me." It was so open and frank, there wasn't hiding from the pain of it all, it was almost like a celebration. It was so powerful to think that someone could go into death that boldly; she was complete at thirty! I think she had a three-year-old, all these reasons that a person could have so many complaints about how things were going. There was a level of faith in things and how they are supposed to go. I remember running to the bathroom crying and crying. I don't know how she came to have that level of faith. Maybe it had something to do with all the love she was receiving, and trusting more in love than in fear.

When someone is dying, most of the time I try to be there every day until the person dies. When someone has a true spiritual path and connection, a real experience, not a heady intellectual concept, it does seem to make a person's death easier for them. I always feel like my job is easier in those cases, too, like something is already rolling, already established. When I worked with AIDS patients in the hospice house it seemed that people who had not had time to come to terms with difficult relationships had less peaceful deaths. I remember one young man whose father came to see him and he said to his dad, "I'm dying here, let's get some things settled," and from my point of view it did make for a more peaceful death for him. So maybe for this woman the combination of a spiritual experience and the loving relationships with friends and family, where it appeared there was no unfinished business, was a big factor in her graceful acceptance and peaceful passing.

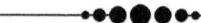

The closer to death someone is, the more subtle my work becomes because there is so much less that needs to be done. If there is a needle required it is just one needle, and I stay attuned to what feedback the body is giving. Sometimes it is apparent that I did too much so when I go back tomorrow I have to be aware of how much the body wants or doesn't want. Trusting the subtle is really hard because you feel like you're not doing anything, but working with the dying gives you that training ground. This is a way of working, i.e. doing less and less as the body begins to shut down in preparation for death as compared to the Western medical model where more and more is done to try to keep the patient alive.

I was working on a patient with pancreatic cancer yesterday, and in the pulse I was feeling the level of chaos her body is in. She's in hospice care now and the prognosis is that she has maybe two months to live. She asked me about a particular type of vitamin therapy that she had heard about for her heart because she had a heart attack last week. She is in a lot of pain and she can't tolerate morphine, so they tried a nerve block for her pain and she had a heart attack. Methadone is the latest thing they have tried and that is going okay, but even that she's not tolerating very well. So here we have a situation where she's really not tolerating the meds at all well, and receiving acupuncture is the one thing that she is saying is actually reducing the pain and giving her some relief.

Feeling that level of instability, feeling just into the heart position, I could feel that there was so much instability there that even a treatment that's particularly for the heart, in this case the vitamin, would be more stressful for her heart, at least for now, because the integrity of the system is going. So I told her "No, no more, it is only putting more stress on an already fragile system that's trying to consolidate." When we start to die things start to separate, so the body, in its attempt to try to live, still attempts to consolidate what is being pushed apart.

This woman is so open to receiving the pulse work and acupuncture, but sometimes you run into a situation where there is conflict about what you may think, what the family may think, versus what the person who is dying may think. I've had people call me and say, "This is exactly what my son or husband or friend needs," and then I meet them and they say, "I don't want anything to do with that; go away, I'm good." I certainly respect what the client wants, but I've found if I can just check their pulse, if there is some kind of contact, I start to form a relationship with them right away that is safe and non-intrusive. Touch is so lacking in medical care now that even a patient's pulse is taken by a machine, so if they will allow the touch of taking the pulse they may be open to more after that.

One of my patients was a woman in a nursing home who had been paralyzed in an automobile accident. Her daughter-in-law called me to see if there was anything I could do to treat her bedsores, so I gave her a treatment and her response was, "I don't think it's doing anything, I don't feel anything." But she called me the next week and said, "You know what? I don't know if it's doing anything for the bed sores, but I felt this peace that none of these pills are giving me, so I want you to come back." With regular treatments the bed sores were better, the peace was there, and she got to the point where she could get back in her wheelchair and she started going to the computer labs.

I got really close to her over those three years and there was no reluctance on her part to show me how she was feeling. There would be some days when she was yelling and furious, days when she was just weeping, and days when we would just talk and talk about whatever; it was wonderful. Then she got pneumonia and she was transferred to intensive care where she was intubated. I went to see her but they wouldn't let me do any acupuncture, so I was asking myself, "What do I do, what do I do?" So I started to do a little more touch and I bought some CDs for her to listen to whenever she wanted. She became very attached to the music and would write notes to me about it, so that was a way for us to stay attached when she couldn't talk. She was scared of death, and bringing the music was one way I hoped that I could help her stay calm. But it also brought up in me how afraid I would be under these circumstances, seeing the look of panic in her eyes because of that tube down her throat, wondering what would bring her some peace, and what would bring me peace if it were me.

The Qigong, the touch, and the acupuncture give so much help when people are afraid. It could be fear about a surgery, about delivering a baby, about dying, almost anything. One of my goals is to help ease that intense fear, some little bit of connection with another being. I think when people can feel connected to something, something higher, or another person or family, something happens and it's very powerful, and yet it's so simple. Basically, having an open heart and being able to connect with somebody where they are, bringing a peaceful presence, and offering a technique helps with their distress. People have offered this to me, so to be able to offer that back, that is really lovely, just to help when things get really, really intense. We will all have those intense times, and just recognizing that, and being present with somebody in it helps them navigate and hopefully have it transform into something else, experience it more fully, and see what's underneath it.

———————————•••••••———————————

Being able to do this is certainly part of my personal journey. When I was working at the hospice house for AIDS patients I would walk out of there at the end of the day feeling like a mess, like I had a hundred and eight things going the wrong direction, and internally there was so much chaos. Over the years, now, it has been a process of accepting each one of those the best that I can, and there is definitely more ability to accept that humanity in me and the fears that I carry. Therapy, Qigong, ballet, Tibetan Buddhism, things that I seek for joy and health, are all ways that help me become more and more aware of me. When someone is talking to me who is dying, or not talking, more and more there's a way that I can understand more about their journey, have empathy, have a recognition that I know that place in me, I know that experience, so it helps me in what I can do in terms of helping that person.

I learned so much about dying and relationships from my hospice patients. When I was helping one young man with his pain he began telling me about his life and all the crazy things he had done, and then he came around to this story about his father. He and his father had always had kind of a rough go of it, and finally, now that he was dying, he addressed their relationship. As I was listening to him I said, "That's similar to the relationship that I have with my dad," and he said, "Talk to your dad, talk to him, why wait?" I will never forget that.

He was one of the patients who were so open to what was happening with them and it seemed like very little was needed from me in those situations. I would take the pulse, do some acupuncture, some Qigong, they would tell me stories about their families, but not too much was needed. I thought about how terrified I would be in their situation but saw that their acceptance, and allowing the experience to be what it was, somehow allowed their pain to ease off; I could just feel things moving.

Another of our patients absolutely hated being sick, and there were days when it almost seemed as if the acupuncture brought out the anger. But I don't even think it was that, I just think it helped him move out of kind of being numb to being more connected to the reality of where he was, like the anger was an honest connection to where he was, and from there he could have moments and a little bit of peace just because he could find some acceptance about his rage. But the worst situation was when he was just totally shut down, refusing his situation, refusing his experience, and that's when I felt that we were the least effective. We would often get yelled at, "Get out of here," and it seemed to me that on the days when he was really shut down, in great resistance to the reality of his situation, the emotional pain created more physical pain and he would need more morphine.

Being able to help someone, whether it is my regular patients who come to me for wellness or people who are close to the end of their lives, is the best part of my job. I wouldn't say that I have a worst or hardest part, only that there are times when I feel limited in my ability to help and wish I had more to offer. Working with the dying pushes me to face my own questions and fears and work through those. I want to be authentic and transparent, honest and open, and one of my draws to working with the dying is that many of them have dropped the defenses that are typically part of our everyday lives, and when they can do that there is something very special that happens, there's a richness, an openness: it's really beautiful.

Aromatherapy/Essential Oils Overview

Application

There is a long list of uses of essential oils that include stress, pain, and anxiety reduction; relaxation, rejuvenation, and beauty care; calming emotions and distressed mental states; feeling more connected spiritually; strengthening the immune system; and treating fungal, bacterial, and viral infections.

In medical settings essential oils are used for all of the above, as well as reducing nausea; helping with sleep problems; easing the fear, sadness, and grief of major life changes; and helping with a peaceful death.

Essential oils are highly concentrated and must be used wisely, requiring the user and/or the aromatherapy practitioner be educated in the beneficial and proper uses as well as the contraindications. Oils can be used in the following ways:

1. Inhaled briefly, a quick whiff. If the reaction to the aroma is negative it is better to choose another oil.
2. Disbursed in a room.
3. Diluted with a carrier oil and applied to the body, often as a hand or foot rub or a small amount directly to the part of the body that is being treated.
4. A small amount disbursed in a bath.
5. Sometimes taken internally, but with caution.

History

There can be no accurate beginning date for the use of botanicals but it is safe to say from archeological data that they have been a part of cultural practices throughout recorded history in religious practices, ceremonies, medicine, and embalming. Hippocrates (c. 460- c. 370) promoted them for daily baths and massage, the *De materia medica* written in the 1st century AD by the Greek Physician Pedanius Dioscorides listed many herbs and essential oils, and they are an important part of Indian ayurvedic medicine said to have been practiced for thousands of years up to the present time. By the 16th century, books were being published on the distillation and uses of essential oils, and in France the results of research on the anti-bacterial properties of essential oils was published in 1888. Rene Maurice-Gattefosse' (1881-1950), was a French chemist and scholar who coined the term "aromatherapy," and published a book by that name in 1937.

In the 19th century much of medicine, particularly in the United States, turned to isolating the active properties of oils to create pharmaceuticals in laboratories. With the increased interest in and use of natural medicines, essential oils are once again being used as alternatives to pharmaceuticals or as part of an integrated treatment plan.

The International Organization for Standardization (ISO) states on their website at www.iso.org that they set specific standards of essential oils, i.e., that an oil contains what it says it does in specified proportions, but does not test for purity or for therapeutic qualities. It is important, therefore, that the consumer and health care professionals do their due diligence and purchase from companies who make full disclosure about their products, including where the raw materials are grown, under what conditions (no herbicides or pesticides), the distillation process, and the purity. Oils that contain additives are not pure and will not produce the desired benefits.

Requirements for licensure or certification

There is no official form of accreditation to become an aromatherapist, although the national education standards for aromatherapists are set by the following:

Alliance of International Aromatherapists (AIA)
www.alliance-aromatherapists.org/
The National Association for Holistic Aromatherapy (NAHA)
https://naha.org/
Aromatherapy Registration Council (ARC)
www.aromatherapycouncil.org/

The AIA lists recognized schools that teach aromatherapy[1], with instructional hours ranging from 100 to 400. The higher levels provide the educational requirements necessary to sit for the Aromatherapy Registration Council's (ARC) registration examination.

Most practitioners use aromatherapy as part of their existing professional practice in the fields of medicine, psychotherapy, massage, energy healing, and/or spas. The licensure and certification requirements for these fields are applicable to the added component of essential oils.

Summary

Odors and aromas are powerful stimuli, evoking an immediate reaction that is experienced as an emotional and a physiological response. The olfactory bulbs are part of the limbic system and directly connect to the areas of the brain that process emotion, memory, and learning.

In understanding how essential oils affect physiology, and therefore health, current research[2] in treating bacterial, viral, and fungal infections, shows four mechanisms:

1. Destroys the harmful cells outright.
2. Interrupts a step in the process of replication so that an illness or condition cannot spread.

3. Blocks the entrance to cells where harmful organisms would have an environment in which they could duplicate, thus preventing damage to the invaded cell and proliferation of the invader.

4. Enhances the curative effects of pharmaceuticals in some cases.

For the individual who wants to use essential oils for self-treatment he or she must understand the uses, benefits, and contraindications for each oil, and purchase high-grade products. By following these guidelines, medical research has shown them to be safe and non-toxic, absent the side effects of pharmaceuticals.

---

1. Note that the American College of Healthcare Sciences, whose president, Dorene Peterson's interview appears below, is the only accredited Alliance of International Aromatherapists' Level II Professional Aromatherapy training program in the United States at the time of this publication.

2. References

National Center for Biotechnology, www.ncbi.nim.nih.gov

National Center for Complementary and Integrative Health, www.nccih.nih.gov

National Center for Biotechnology Information, www.ncbi.nim.nih.gov

Aromatherapist Interview

Dorene Petersen
Bachelor of Arts in Social Anthropology and Archeology
Naturopath
Acupuncturist
President and CEO of the American College of
Healthcare Sciences, Portland, Oregon

Introduction

Many of the nurses that I interviewed use essential oils as part of their patient care, and I wanted to find someone whom I would consider an expert on the history, research, manufacturing processes, uses, and outcomes of their use. I was fortunate to find Dorene Petersen, President, Principal, and CEO of the American College of Healthcare Sciences in Portland, Oregon.

The college is accredited by the Distance Education and Training Council and Council for Higher Education Accreditation. Specializing in holistic health, courses are offered in aromatherapy, herbal medicine, holistic nutrition, and anatomy and physiology. With students in over 70 countries throughout the world, it provides CE credits for pharmacists, naturopaths, and veterinarians, and CEUs for registered nurses and licensed massage therapists.

Interview

What I do here is oversee the day-to-day strategies and direction of the college. I also work a lot with the curriculum, not just to insure the factual credibility of the curriculum, but also to insure that my particular philosophy, which is very holistic, is built into it.

I am involved in consulting and liaison with leaders in the natural health industry, including consulting on product formulations and advising on emerging markets. I travel a lot to look at the growing and production sites of the materials that we use in our essential oils, and to investigate emerging international markets for holistic health products including Greece, Jamaica, Belize, Nicaragua, Indonesia, China, Paraguay, Korea, Japan, and Singapore.

My interest in holistic health started when I was very young, being heavily influenced as a child growing up in New Zealand by my parents and grandparents who focused on a healthy lifestyle, wellness, organic gardening, and harvesting local wild crops like berries and mushrooms. I can recall going out mushrooming in the early morning, picking berries, gathering seeds for the garden, gathering horse poop for the garden, helping my dad make manure tea and things like that to spray on the plants. I helped my grandmother gather dandelions and yellow dock and make the tinctures and decoctions to make medicines for the winter.

I was really interested in ethnobotany and culture, people's perception of wellness and ill health, and how people's perception of that was different in different cultures. In 1973 I graduated from the University of Otago in Dunedin, New Zealand with a Bachelor of Arts in Social Anthropology & Archeology with a focus on ethnobotany and traditional medicine.

When I left University from that first degree I married, had two children, divorced, and started working as a medical social worker to support myself and my children. In the region where I worked I had two wonderful mentors and teachers, and my primary responsibilities were working with elderly people and people who were coming towards the end of their life but still out in the community. My goal was to keep them in the community and living at home as long as they could, but I found that after doing that job for a year or so I just felt like I was cleaning up the flotsam and the jetsam of society. There weren't enough resources for these people, and when it became too much for society the elderly just became a problem and then it became my duty to tidy them up and put them somewhere where they weren't so much of a problem.

I didn't care for that. The services that were available to me to provide to the elderly were, in my opinion, not based on wellness protocols. The meals were really inadequate and lacking in nutrition, heavily cooked, heavily salted, heavily sugared, and very few fresh vegetables. This disturbed me because I am a great believer in you are what you eat.

A lot of what I saw in these elderly people was that they were actually not sick in themselves, but a lot of the symptoms were from other drugs they were taking, and a lot of the drugs they were taking were for physical issues that were a direct result of their accumulated lifestyle over the years. So it really opened my eyes to what eventually became my mantra, which is, "Wellness is something that happens every day." It's not something you do once a month, it's every little thing you do every day that produces wellness and it is cumulative. The reverse is true, as well.

I became very interested in this wellness approach, so I went to the South Pacific College of Natural Therapy in Aukland which was a four-year training to become a naturopathic doctor. It's different than the training here in the States, so it's based more on a wellness protocol. We were taught all of the modalities; we learned acupressure, massage, homeopathy, color therapy, nutrition, herbal medicine, aromatherapy, and kinesiology. Many of my teachers were naturopaths with years of experience and they taught me so much, including opening my eyes to the power of word, touch, color, intention, visualization, and individualization. After I graduated I practiced for quite a few years, and those were the tenants of my naturopathic practice.

While I was still in college, in my second year, I had been asked to set up an extramural department; in those days that was the name for correspondence courses. In New Zealand and Australia extramural correspondence was a big deal, particularly in Australia because it's a huge country, and they wanted it set up just in herbal medicine so I began preparing the curriculum. Because I had my life training from the time I was a child and read a lot, and I was learning the specifics at college, I had more background than some of the other students, so that was terrific. It was a salaried position and I was very happy doing that, I enjoyed it, and we had a number of students working in that department toward their degree through distance learning. Of course in those days it was all papers and post office and everything was hard copy in color-coded files.

After a couple of years, just before I graduated, they let me know they were trying to get accredited by an osteopathic group out of England, and that organization preferred not to have an extramural department and they wouldn't accredit it. So I was told that the program I was heading was going to be closed down, but they said, "It's really your department, you've done all the work, we want you to have it. So you can run it, teach out the students you're teaching, and then we'll no longer offer the course." My initial thought was, "Oh, okay, I think I just lost my job." But then it was, "I'm gong to take care of these students;" that was my primary focus, to insure the students weren't compromised, and that is really the foundation for this school, the American College of Healthcare Sciences.

Before long I was running my clinic, doing the extramural course, and had to hire two or three people to help me run everything while I still did my clinic. Eventually I got to the place where I was more interested in educating people how to be well, educating others to educate others how to be well. I thought it had more scope than me just sitting with someone one-on-one as a naturopath, even though I really enjoyed that and I had some very interesting patients and some good results.

I did find that with the modalities that I had studied and trained with for my naturopathic degree, I didn't have a modality that gave immediate results to someone. Even then, back in the early 1980s, there was the mentality of "take a pill, get better." "Put this on the owie and the owie goes away." Insuring compliance, and also wanting someone to walk out of the clinic feeling better, because of course that was my desire, that somebody would feel better, I went to Hong

Kong to study acupuncture, and that gave me what I was looking for, a way to help somebody right away. I learned the minimum needling technique, that was very interesting, and I saw some quite miraculous work in China while I was studying there and that really opened my eyes again.

The minimal needling technique is a technique that is based on the theory that there are master points in your body that, if the chi is blocked and you needle those points correctly, either with a stimulating or a sedating point, depending on the symptom picture, it can clear the entire channel. So rather than putting many needles in somebody along the entire channel, or along a meridian, just needle these very specific points; you might only insert three needles.

I saw some amazing things in China and learned a lot from the doctor I took my training with. I learned intra-vertebra needling where tiny needles are placed horizontally along the spine and taped in place to work with the nervous system, the nerves radiating out from the spine that were associated with whatever issue was going on. The needles don't go in very deep, just enough to create some stimulation or sedation, and might be left in for as long as a week. I thought it was a particularly successful technique: it was less invasive for the client, it took less time, and it certainly got results, I saw some amazing results. Ear needling, moxibustion, Qigong energy healing, surgery with no anesthesia done with the patient wide awake getting electric current through acupuncture needles – these are some of the things that I saw in China that just blew my mind.

One of the things that I did in New Zealand was to travel around giving face-to-face workshops and trainings with students throughout the country, as well as doing the distance learning. During that time I saw a lot of land that had previously been used for growing tobacco just lying unused, huge drying sheds completely unused, and the farmers going broke. I thought it would be great if they grew herbs, did essential oils, turned a building into a distillery and another into a drying room. When my program was flourishing in New Zealand, I wanted to be able to provide my students with quality essential oils so that they could learn experientially by using herbs and oils in their own healing. Finding really high quality therapeutic raw material was a real challenge back then. There was very little certified organic, very few essential oils that weren't adulterated, and of course, working in a busy clinic I became acutely aware that the results of the wellness work is sometimes only as good as the quality of the product.

I talked to a few farmers and it became evident that the farmers really didn't have the training or the education necessary to raise the plants for the oils. At that time there was a government organization in New Zealand called the Department of Scientific and Industrial Research, where farmers could call up and get information and training. So I went through them and they asked me how I was going to find the experts. I said that I really didn't know but that I was sure I could find a way. I told them it would create a great trade, we could be exporting, because there are few raw materials available right now in the world. So that's what I did, I applied to the New Zealand Development Board for a grant to travel to seek out and interview the experts and was awarded $150,000.00. My husband, Robert, was one of the experts that I brought back to New Zealand to teach distillation; that's how I met him and that's how I ended up in the United States about five years later and started the college in 1978.

We created a series of teaching workshops throughout New Zealand in which he trained people, not to just distill but to design and manufacture the stills because the design and the efficiency of the equipment is a very integral part of the success of distillation, it can affect the therapeutic quality of the oils. Lavender is being distilled there now, really great lavender, really great tea tree oil, and several others. At that time I didn't expand it to the point where we had our own product line, I was just more interested in creating education for a group of people that were really at the mercy of the Japanese who had contracted the leases to grow the tobacco and then they said, "No, we don't want it any more," so the farmers were left up in the air. With growing the raw materials and distilling the oils it's a good industry now, and people were able to maintain their livelihood, so it worked out well.

I now have my own line of oils for the apothecary, we call it the apothecary shop oils, they're all the oils the students get. My primary focus is that they are certified organic. I'm a great believer in certified organic, not just for the quality of the end product, but for the larger picture of when we do business we want it to be sustainable, we want to be taking care of the planet and the people who produce the raw materials.

I travel all over the world and I visit all my vendors to make sure that what we're getting is what they say it is as far as fair trade and sustainability, and is organic. I've seen enough examples to know that you can't always trust what you are being told. For instance, in Turkey I've seen women who are harvesting rows of roses, which have to be harvested in the very early hours of the morning to get the flower at the peak where the essential oil is ready to distill, working on a hillside that is just littered with cans of spent herbicide and pesticide. A lot of the women were ill, a lot of the women had cancer, they didn't even know what they were picking the roses for, didn't know they were being made into essential oils. It was a real eye opener for me. I had been buying from this distillery and they had been saying - it was before the days of certified organic where everything had to be credentialed - they were saying that yes, it's all natural, and no, we don't use any chemicals, but of course they were just lying.

But the very worst thing at this particular distillery was, and the other thing I'm always concerned about, is what they do with spent material because there is a lot of waste produced from essential oil production. There is very hot water that comes from the stove that has some residual oil in it and other aromatic materials, and then there is also all of the plant material, left over plant material that either has to be composted or gotten rid of in some way. You'll see throughout France, throughout the lavender region, huge mounds in the fields of spent lavender which takes a long time to break down.

Some innovative distillers are doing things like making paper, making straw bales, some crops you can feed to animals as animal feed, and that's great, too, because it can improve the health of the animal, but you can't do that with lavender. So I was particularly interested in what this one rose distillery was doing with the spent material and they told me, "Oh, we take care of the hydrosols," the hot liquid that comes from the distill, "we pipe that to the local village and the women use it to do their washing." I thought, "Well, isn't that nice." So I get to the distillery and I can really smell the essential oil and I'm thinking, "If that is coming from the distillery they're losing a lot of volatile material, which is expensive;" it didn't make sense to me.

So during the lunch break I went for a walk, it's a huge distillery, I walked outside, across the road, through the trees and bushes in this rural area, because I was smelling it stronger and stronger. Sure enough, there's the pipe emptying into the river, and sure enough the water was black, dead, slime, dying fish. They were heating the river up, killing the river, and I gave the head of that place what-for. I never did business with them again, and they could not have cared less. They simply dismissed me, my voice was irrelevant to them, but at least I felt better about making a stand and also trying to educate them on the long-term effects of what they were doing and how what they were doing would be way more detrimental down the road than they could even imagine. Let's hope it's not like that anymore.

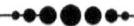

So that is my focus with my essential oils. All of our oils are tested so I'm sure they're not contaminated with anything. If I have any doubt at all I run them through pesticide tests, and all of that is very expensive. We buy very small batches which the students use in their courses and which we sell in our store at the college.

Testing essential oils for purity and potency is a very technical process so a customer has to rely on the person or company that is buying and reselling it. The popular multi-level marketing companies have done a lot to improve awareness of essential oils, availability, and potential of the oils, so in that sense I think they've done a great service to the profession and to the industry. They've certainly increased usage of essential oils, and I'm sure from the distiller's point of view it's terrific because distilleries that may not have been able to sell the oils now have contracts for the next ten years, so it's really created a great boost for the industry.

So I'm happy in that regard, but unfortunately, when they teach their sales people to provide advice, particularly advice on how to administer oils, it's not accurate and it's not based on what is believed to be general safety practices. For example, somebody might drop thyme oil directly on somebody's spine and various other locations on the body and it will blister the skin, thyme oil will blister. Of course this is not a desirable result, damaging, completely unacceptable, and that puts the entire industry at risk and the profession at risk. What the practitioners are told to say is that it's the toxins coming out of the body that creates the blistering. It's impossible for toxins to come out of the body through a blister when you burn the skin, it's just silly, so it makes me rather cross.

So when you're searching for an essential oil how do you know that the information you are getting is accurate? Go for the Latin names if possible. I'll give you an example, lavender. The lavender you want to use is lavandula angustifolia. There is another lavender called lavandin, it's lavendula intermedia, which contains camphor, which is a stimulant. Lavendula angustifolia contains no camphor, and it is a sedative. Most people think of lavender as a sedative, but if they buy lavender and it's not labeled with the Latin name they could end up with lavandin and it's not going to add to the sedative effect.

There are other considerations when using essential oils, and these are the things that we teach in the college for students who are studying to become aromatherapists. As soon as you inhale an oil you have a physiological reaction: your hypothalamus is stimulated, the oil enters your blood stream through the olfactory bulb, and the endocrine system is going to be flooded with a cascade of something, depending on the oil. This physiological reaction is going to occur even if you can't smell it, maybe you have a cold, it doesn't matter, it's still going to happen. You don't have to have a physical interpretation of the smell in order to have a physiological reaction. However, at the same time, you're having a psychological reaction. There are very few things, when you think about it, that give you both physiological and psychological reactions simultaneously; that's what I think is so intriguing about aromatherapy. That's where the subjectivity comes in, because there are a lot of things that can affect it.

When you're working with a person you would look at the goal you're trying to achieve and you would then come up with a selection. In our teachings here, in both the master's and associates program, and the certificates and diplomas, the aromatherapists get taught that you should be able to select about seven oils, it doesn't have to be a huge number, it could be less than seven, but start with about seven. As you are assembling your oils you are thinking about the constituents within the oil and the results that that oil will produce because of those constituents, so it's a very straightforward connection. You're also thinking about the synergy between any oils you might put together. Some oils really work well together, some oils work better alone. So you're thinking about the synergy of what you might put together and then, if you're working face to face with somebody, you would work on more of the psychological, emotional component. You would either have the client smell the oil with a strip, and you're just really reviewing what that means for the client, and allow that person to tell you if they like it or not. They wouldn't have to say why they did or did not like it because they might actually not recall why or why not. Because the aroma of the oil goes straight to the limbic system it might open up a flood of memories, the memories themselves might not arise as a memory but as a fight or flight response in the body, it could create a stress response, so all the client is feeling is stress even though the oil may be one that typically calms a person.

The intriguing thing about olfaction is that the memory of the first time you ever smelled a particular aroma is retained and that's the way you respond for the rest of your life. You can override a negative reaction but it's not a good idea if you're trying to achieve wellness. Eventually the memory can come back, and that's why it's so good for working with psychological and emotional problems. Sometimes it can unlock something and the person can have a real healing that way, and that's great.

But here's another thing that can happen, conditioning. Say, for example, that a person has to fly to a lot of places for business and that person is very anxious about flying. They have heard that lavender will help calm people in such situations so now they use lavender every time they fly, and even though it helps some they still have a lot of anxiety about flying. Eventually, every time that person smells lavender it provokes a feeling of anxiety because they have become conditioned to the pairing of the events, anxiety and the aroma of lavender, so it comes to have the opposite effect than intended. In our college we teach these things, the relationships between personal history and the emotional and psychological links to the olfactory stimulus.

It is also important to know a lot about anatomy and physiology, you have to really understand the pathway of an oil through the body, whether it's going to be eliminated through the kidneys, the liver, or the lungs. If somebody is compromised, is on a lot of drugs, you have to be careful because the body is already dealing with pathways that are blocked, like gridlock on the freeway. In this case you don't want to add more to the blockage by laying on constituents that the body is having to eliminate. You don't want to use oils with a lot of phenols if somebody has kidney issues, for example, so there is a lot to learn.

In chronic illness and end-of-life care there are certain oils that have been found in research studies to be effective in easing physical and emotional issues.[1] Lavender is used to ease anxiety and with Altzheimer's patients. In a 2008 study with fifty-eight hospice patients bergamot was used, an oil that is very uplifting for people suffering from depression, for people who are really low and don't have the capability of seeing anything good happening. Frankincense and lavender as a blend was used for a hand massage and people reported less pain and less depression. No tests were done on the separate oils so it's hard to know if one was better than the other, but that particular blend seemed to be extremely effective. Jasmine is also used for depression, and when it was applied topically to the abdomen, breathing rate, blood oxygen saturation, and systolic and diastolic pressure all indicated a quickening and arousal, so there was definitely stimulation and activation: it just generally uplifts people when they are in a sad state.

Rose is another one that's really good for both pain and depression. It is excellent for a lot of pain states, including the pain of childbirth, so a person in pain might want to try rose essential oil. For nausea, any of the mints, spearmint, peppermint, they're all excellent, and lemon, lemon is another great one. You can make ice cubes from these, just one drop of the essential oil in an ice cube, and if a patient is not doing well and can't take much nourishment, sucking on a small ice cube can sometimes bring huge relief. Ravensara, which has an aromatic resemblance to eucalyptus, has mentholated and clarifying characteristics and can give a lot of comfort to people. If I were a nurse I might try one or more of these oils, depending upon the need, and just monitor very closely to make sure my patient was not having a bad experience with any of them.

Homeopathic remedies are also helpful: aspen for a sense of foreboding and a fear that can't be named; mimulus for a known fear; arnica Montana for mental strain or shock; aconite for extreme mental tension and fear of death; and arsenica for restlessness, anxiety, and fear. As a practitioner I think about it as drawing on arrows for your bow, or tools in your toolbox, to find what will be of the greatest help.

I also know that energy in the room can have a huge impact on your physical, mental, and emotional wellbeing, so it's important from a holistic standpoint to not just provide comfort to the client, but also you want to keep the room clear which essential oils and color can help with.

I haven't seen many people dying, but when I was working as a medical social worker I did work with people who were in enormous amounts of pain because of arthritis, who were emitting bitterness from every pore, and anger, and you just wish nothing for them but a quiet, relaxed death because they are so anguished. One of my patients was a woman who had such terrible arthritis that she was bedridden so I would do home visits. She was so angry that when she spoke she would almost spit her words out; she had so much hostility and anxiety and upset.

I can remember when I first went to see her I could barely get two feet from the bed; I just felt this huge wall of black energy surrounding this person. So I did a lot of essential oils in the room, a lot of color, I would always bring her flowers, a lot of visualization and mentally clearing a space for her. Eventually, I was able to sit on the bed, but for a long time she didn't want me anywhere near, was afraid that I would bump the bed because it created such agony for her. I worked with the doctor to give her pain medication to the increased level where it should have been all along; it was woefully inadequate, she was in agony. I'm a great believer that nobody should be in pain. I mean, I'm a naturopath and I believe in natural remedies, but if somebody's in pain bring on the drugs. It was the withdrawal of morphine that caused my dad's death.

When I would see my arthritis patient I would give her a sip of water with essences, bring flowers, and she got to the point where I could sit on the bed but she never recovered, she died, but at least there was a little easing. When I first went to see her I was just so shocked at the level of anger and bitterness coming from this person and that it could create this, like smoke, almost. You couldn't see it but you could feel it, it was thick, a thickness, like a sticky, thick, black hovering over her being. It almost felt like the room was, I don't want to use the word possessed, but it almost felt like there was something in the room, like an entity.

The other thing I used was sound. I have a beautiful little pair of Tibetan bells that I just gently tap against each other and it makes a beautiful ringing sound. It creates a vibration that seems to cut through, and you can put it on your body and you can just feel the tension going from your body, there is so much relief. All these things can help somebody ease gently into that good death, as they say. I can't imagine anything worse than dying anguished and frightened and in pain.

My father had a particularly difficult death. He had bowel cancer and they said he would last for three months; he lived for four years. That gave me a really interesting one-on-one appreciation for the fact that you just don't know how you're going to be, or how anybody is going to be when it comes to the end of life. My father had a morphine pump but he would still get breakthrough pain sometimes and it was just agonizing for him. He said to me, "You know, Dorene, I always thought if I got to this stage I would want someone to give me a morphine overdose, just end it, but you know, even if I had five minutes pain-free and I would get to see you and your Mom and your sister it would be worth it." So you just never know how you're going to be.

I did what I could for him to keep him comfortable: I used essential oils, I would bathe his feet with water and the eucalyptus and the oils that have that lovely clearing effect, I had diffuses going in his room with clearing oils, and I used a lot of color therapy. I would buy scarves of block colors and drape them on his body and tie a bright orange scarf around his neck and drape it all down the front of his body, and wrap a nice bright scarf around his tummy. All of those things he said really helped.

I also attribute my dad living so much longer than the prognosis to my mother's incredibly good care. She is a nurse, was a matron of a hospital, so she had many years of experience and knew what she was doing. A nurse was coming to the house to help with my father's care and one day she wanted him to go to the hospital for some tests. My mother did not think it was a good idea, but my dad said, "Well, maybe it will give you a break. I'll just go down there for two or three days and I'll be back." He had his morphine pump with him but when the morphine ran out they couldn't get any more because it was locked in a cupboard and the only nurse who had access to it was at lunch, so within an hour my father went into severe pain and deep shock and died. My mother said he had an absolutely agonizing death. Nobody should have to die that way. She was dreadfully upset about it as we all were.

My mother and I have talked about death and dying over the years, she's seen many of her patients die and would sit with them and hold their hands. She's really great to talk to, and I have asked her what happens when somebody dies? She said she's seen a spirit, it starts from the feet and it just completely goes up and leaves the body. She said it's such an amazing thing to see, and it's such a relief for the person that once the spirit is gone the body is dead. We were lucky that we got to speak to Dad at length about his death, how he felt about it, if he was scared. He said, "Don't worry, I'm still going to be around you," and I said, "How will I know that you are?" "Whenever you hear a strange bird, that will be me." Since that day I believe my father has come to me more than once, because I've been in certain locations and I'll hear a bird call which is completely unrelated to the surroundings and I'll be like, "Hi Dad."

I was also fortunate as a child to grow up with an aunt who was not so much religious as spiritual, and when I would ask her about dying she would say to me, "You don't want to worry about dying. Dying is like opening a door and you walk through it, and everyone you ever knew is there." So I said, "Okay, that sounds pretty good." And she said, "Even people you knew in another life, not even in this life," and I said, "Okay, jolly good." I believed her, I still do. So that's nice for me personally, but people who have anxiety and can't let go, any of the essential oils that are clearing, any of the eucalyptol, the ravensara, frankincense, might be helpful: when you inhale them it gives a clarity, maybe helps clear the way, helps you see the path that you are to take and opens that door.

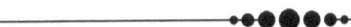

So these are some of my experiences with wellness protocols, which brings me back to the college. We hire our faculty very carefully, after numerous interviews, not just looking at their credentials and what their clinical work has been, but we also look at their emotional intelligence, psychological intelligence, their capacity for caring and empathy. These are really important qualities for anyone who is going to be working in the wellness arena that we're working in.

So I would say that this is the most difficult part of my job now, training graduates in such a way that they have the awareness that each person they will be working with is a unique and wonderful human being, to meet each person where they are, and to work with them from that perspective. I feel anxious sometimes, I feel very responsible putting people out there to work one-on-one to achieve wellness. We're always trying to build that appreciation for the individual into our teaching, to put your own judgment and your own opinion aside, and just work with them where they are. It's no good, for example, to take somebody who is smoking twenty cigarettes a day, eating three big macs and drinking coke and putting them on a juice fast.

The best part of my job is that I've got fabulous staff who have been here with me a long time, who embrace the mission and vision of what we're doing, and who are really committed to wellness, not just wellness for themselves individually but wellness within the college, wellness between all of us, and extending that out into the world.

Another wonderful part of my job is having successful graduates. You just need to go on our website at www.achs.edu to see our outstanding alumni who are doing amazing things in their lives and really helping people. Many of the books in our store here are written by our graduates. We have members of the military who have come out of the service and helped themselves through Post Traumatic Stress Disorder (PTSD) and are now helping others. We've had active duty students who have received their assignments and their kits in their tents in Bahrain. There are great stories of success, wellness, and prosperity, so that gives us a huge sense of achievement. We currently have students in eighty different countries, so I just like to think that we are sort of a beacon of wellness in the world, spreading wellness worldwide. Check out our Facebook page to see more about our work.

I'm a great believer in if you're well, if you're educated, and you've got a full tummy, you're dry and cozy at night and your kids are alright, then pretty much life is good. That's what any of us want, it's no mystery. If we can achieve that then I think there will be genuinely happier communities, not just within our immediate sphere but worldwide. So whenever I travel I am always looking at ways I can enhance people's lives wherever I am. Recently I met with a company in Africa that is interested in oils. They teach people there how to make soap, and for every bar of soap they sell they give one away. Hygiene is really poor there, and a lot of the children have illnesses because of it, so this is a great service to the community.

I feel very fortunate that I've had the influences and the opportunities in life that I've had, and the blessings that I have now. I adore my grandchildren and spend a lot of time with them, I have wonderful friends whom I do things with, I stay physically active, I play the piano every chance I get, I have a wonderfully supportive husband, and I practice gratitude. Every morning when I wake up I spend five minutes practicing gratitude even if I don't feel it in that particular morning. I teach all my staff and my family to practice gratitude, and I smile at everybody I pass in the street. Gratitude for what we have, connecting to others with a smile; small things, maybe, but they are powerful and make a difference in the world.

---

1. Chang, S.Y. (2008). Effects of aroma hand massage on pain, state anxiety and depression in hospice patients with terminal cancer. Taehan Kanho Hakhoe Chi., 38(4):493-502.
From: http://info.achs.edu/blog/depression-and-anxiety-can-essential-oils-help

Music Therapy Overview

Application

Music therapy is used for pain relief, anxiety reduction, calming of agitation, and promoting sleep. For Alzheimer and nursing home patients it helps them communicate better, helps memory recall, and aids in increasing other cognitive and physical functions such as being more steady on their feet. When patients are active participants in the music therapy, such as group singing or drumming, bonding with their fellow participants occurs and their level of happiness increases. Whether you are a patient in the hospital, in an assisted living center, in a nursing home or adult foster care home, in an Alzheimer's care center, or living at home with assistance, if your treatment plan involves music therapy it is obvious from the above-list how it may provide significant benefits to a better quality of life.

History

It seems safe to say that using tones and rhythm in one form or another is as old as mankind. No matter what culture one explores you see and hear music as entertainment, a way to affect mood, a means of physical relaxation or stimulation, and a means to bring people together in a shared experience.

In the King James version of the Bible, I Samuel 16:14-23, a musician was sent for when "an evil spirit from God" was tormenting Saul. " . . .Saul was refreshed, and was well, and the evil spirit departed from him," but only temporarily it should be noted. Today the evil spirit would probably be diagnosed as a mental illness, possibly a severe biochemical imbalance, and Saul would be prescribed music as an adjunct to other treatments, not as the only treatment. This is how music therapy is used today, as an important component in a multidimensional treatment plan.

All of these uses, throughout all the cultures over all the centuries provide the foundation for modern music therapy. During and after World Wars I and II, volunteers went into Veterans' hospitals to play for the wounded soldiers. Hospital staff noted the positive reactions of the patients and the musicians recognized that they needed more training in using music as medicine. As a result, several music therapy associations were founded but were short-lived until The National Association for Music Therapy was founded in 1950, followed by The American Association for Music Therapy in 1971. In 1998 these two associations merged with the new name of the American Music Therapy Association (AMTA).

Requirements for certification

Sixty schools offer degrees in music therapy, and currently there are over 5,000 therapists in over 30 countries who hold the credential of Music Therapist-Board Certified (MT-BC). In order to achieve this status, the education, training, and internship requirements are rigorous. The Certification Board for Music Therapists (CBMT) was incorporated in 1983 and has been fully accredited by the National Commission for Certifying Agencies (NCCA) since 1986.

The following description is from http://www.musictherapy.org/about/requirements/

"A professional music therapist holds a bachelor's degree or higher in music therapy from one of over 70 American Music Therapy Association (AMTA) approved college and university programs. The curriculum for the bachelor's degree is designed to impart entry level competencies in three main areas: musical foundations, clinical foundations, and music therapy foundations and principles as specified in the AMTA Professional Competencies. In addition to the academic coursework, the bachelor's degree requires 1200 hours of clinical training, including a supervised internship. Graduate degrees in Music Therapy focus on advanced clinical practice and research.

Upon completion of the bachelor's degree, music therapists are eligible to sit for the national board certification exam to obtain the credential MT-BC (Music Therapist - Board Certified) which is necessary for professional practice. The credential MT-BC is granted by a separate, accredited organization, the Certification Board for Music Therapists (CBMT) www.cbmt.org, to identify music therapists who have demonstrated the knowledge, skills and abilities necessary to practice at the current level of the profession. The purpose of board certification in music therapy is to provide an objective national standard that can be used as a measure of professionalism by interested agencies, groups, and individuals.

In addition, music therapists who currently hold the professional designations of ACMT, CMT or RMT are listed on the National Music Therapy Registry (NMTR) and are qualified to practice music therapy.

Music therapist must meet and practice the Scope of Music Therapy Practice guidelines, the Standards of Clinical Practice, The Code of Ethics, and the Professional Competencies."

Summary

Even if one is not a participant in a treatment plan, listening to, playing, and/or composing music is therapeutic. Performers are often told that their music and the lyrics to their songs helped someone get through a challenging time in their life. Music is used to elevate one's mood and increase one's energy and stamina while working or exercising. Love songs, protest songs, music for ceremonies, lullabies – it seems almost impossible to name an aspect of life that does not include music.

Music Therapist Interview

Gabe
Music Therapist – Board Certified

Introduction

Gabe is a music therapist for Seasons, a hospice and palliative care company that has at the time of the interview twenty six locations across the United States and is the number one employer of music therapists. He is a graduate of the Berklee College of Music in Boston, MA.

Interview

I explain music therapy as an evidence-based practice utilizing music and psychotherapeutic interventions, musical in nature, to achieve non-musical outcomes. We use patient-preferred music rather than a pre-planned musical set because it is much more effective in achieving those non-music outcomes. To explain this further I will describe what I do when I become part of a patient's treatment team.

The first thing I do after getting a referral from a nurse or a healthcare consultant is to schedule a home visit or go to the assisted living facility to conduct a music therapy assessment with the patient. The music therapy assessment consists of music preferences, family dynamics, we assess their spiritual community, and note if they've ever been involved in playing music with others, if they've ever danced or sang, and if they've ever taught music. Based on this I get a feel for who this person is as a whole person, not just as a person who has a terminal illness with only a few months to live. I know what their diagnosis is, I may know about a few of the problems they are having socially, and how they are coping with the death and dying process. So when I go to see them we talk about music, what that means for them, we talk about family and what that means for them, their spirituality, and from there I can craft my goals for our time together.

Some of what I do sounds like what a social worker does. For example, I not only work with the patients, I also work with their families, sometimes just one family member and at other times the whole family. When I meet with the patient for the first time I ask, "Who do you see on a regular basis? Who comes to visit you? Who have you lived with? Who lives nearby?" I get a sense of who is in their lives, and at that point I can ask more specific questions about relationships with various family members so I can get a feel for what their family life might be like these days and what their support system is. All of this information helps me know more about how I can individualize the goals of the music therapy and our relationship, and it gives me insight into how I might be able to relate to family members and who in the interdisciplinary team may need to be included in the conversations. Our teams consist of the doctor, the medical director, nurses, aides, social workers, chaplains, and me, the music therapist.

When I refer to achieving non-musical outcomes, what I mean is that I use music to help the patient achieve a deeper sense of wellbeing. I do an intervention called the iso principle, which is meeting the patient where they're at in order to bring them to a more ideal place. So if a patient is agitated, the music may sound quite agitated, it might not sound pretty at all, but the whole idea is to meet them at that level in order to gradually bring them to a new place. So if it's agitation, we'll meet them by playing rough, maybe staccato, maybe a little loud, maybe a little arrhythmic, maybe even atonal, and then gradually bring all those elements back, gradually introduce some tonality, gradually introduce some more predictable meter. It can look as simple as playing music to the rhythm of their breathing, or their heart rate, so if their heart rate is particularly high, or their breathing rapid and labored, we meet them at that level and then gradually reduce the tempo to entrain them to that slower, calmer rhythm.

Becoming a music therapist is not what I set out to do but when I learned about it I thought that it sounded like a perfect match for me. I've always been a musician since I was a kid; I played trumpet in jazz and blues bands with a lot of musicians in my home town, I played in community bands, and my mentor always taught with an emphasis on giving back to the community.

I had a very musical upbringing but when I went to college I initially decided to go a social work route, so I studied math and science and all the other core curriculum. But at a certain point I felt music calling me back, and after a particularly tumultuous point in my life I decided to make that change and study music. I applied to Berklee College of Music in Boston on a whim and was actually fortunate enough to receive a decent sized scholarship. I first found out about music therapy there, it was a newer program, and I immediately became interested in it. It was a combination of all the things I was interested in – music, science, and helping others, so it was a really good fit for me.

Getting a degree as a music therapist requires four years of study, followed by field placements under the supervision of a music therapist. In Philadelphia, where I was an intern, Seasons has an inpatient and outpatient program. I spent about half my time doing inpatient music therapy and the other half doing patient visits elsewhere. When an opening became available on the West Coast, which is where I am from and where my family lives, I jumped at the chance and am very happy to be back. One big reason is that working with people who are dying has allowed me to see and acknowledge the significance of my loved ones, my family and my friends, and I am grateful to be back with them. I realize that they are going to be the ones who are my companions at the end of life, they will be the ones who will help me through those times. The one thing that I know for sure, that we all die, is still shrouded in mystery, and the best way to set myself up for that time is to have my relationships in good standing with the people who are closest to me in my life.

This is also part of my self-care, spending time with the people who are the most meaningful in my life. On the weekends I like to explore new places, I like to spend time in nature, I find nature particularly grounding and rejuvenating, and I find that so many people at the end of life state that if they have a regret it is that they didn't do all the things they wish they would have. So I take that to heart and really try to be there for my friends and family, to be open to their influence, and to be open to being rejuvenated by the world. Sometimes it's really easy for me to become more guarded and have boundaries that are too high or too thick or too long, so sharing my time with people I love is very important, and being sure not to close myself off to the things in my life that are beautiful and worth taking a moment to enjoy.

In my experience with hospice work, if anything, the people whom I have served have almost given me a sense of looking at the world through rose colored glasses because with so many of them they so desperately crave love and affection, they crave the intimacy of just being with another person who is not going to look at them or treat them in an analytical way. They tell me about all the joys in life as well as all their troubles and strife, but they make a point of mentioning all the good things they have experienced and that gives me a lot of hope and courage to go on in life and take advantage of all the good things that come my way. As the saying goes, "we die the way we lived," and I would like to deposit as many wonderful, positive experiences into my experience bank so that when my day comes I have a beautiful life to look back on.

In order to live my life like this I have to deal with the hardest part of my job, which is to leave my work and not take it home with me. The first thing I do after my last patient of the day is turn my cell phone off, turn my computer off, and not look at my work until the following morning. This takes self-discipline because we get updates twenty-four hours a day on the status of our patients. We get triage reports, we get census reports, there is an endless barrage of information that comes at you twenty-four hours a day, seven days a week, in this line of work. It is so important to strictly follow my designated work schedule because it is very easy to get wrapped up in it and unless I take care of myself I can't be fully present to take care of others the way I want to.

That's the most difficult part of my job, and the best part is being able to honor life by bringing light into the lives of my patients and their families. Often I find that people distance themselves from the dying, maybe because of their own fear of death, and it can be so comforting and even therapeutic to celebrate life in those times and to provide companionship. People don't have to let me into their lives but they allow me in, and it's incredibly humbling and gives me a sense of honor, gratitude, and appreciation.

One day I was referred to visit a woman who was with our hospice because of cancer and at first she did not want to see me because when she heard the words music therapy she thought, "Oh boy, I don't want to hear any harps in my room, I don't want to hear angel music, that's just not the way I want to go." With this information in mind I came into the room without any instruments and I just told her I wanted to sit with her and talk for awhile. She was okay with that. So after gathering as much information as I could regarding the music therapy assessment I came back later that day with my guitar and she allowed me to play some of her favorite music.

We had a really good time together, we laughed, she told me some jokes, I told her some jokes, and we were companions that day. That was a Friday, and when I came in the following Monday she had taken a steep decline. She was no longer verbal and was pretty stuporous lying in her hospital bed. I started playing some soothing music, some clinical improvisation which is usually just soothing chords arpeggiated on the guitar and some humming, just something to aid rest and relaxation.

Her older sister arrived, we met each other and had a brief conversation, I asked her if she would like some time alone with her sister and she said she would, and she spent about ten minutes with her sister in the room. When she came out she asked if I would play another song for them and I said, "Of course, it would be my pleasure."

So I went into the room and started playing "Moon River" by Irving Berlin, which was a favorite of those two as kids, a song their mother used to sing to them. I played the song and after the final chorus I continued to play the cord progression on the guitar just to provide some soothing background music. The sister started talking to the patient saying, "I'm here, I'm with you. I love you, you have friends and family around." She mentioned that there was music in the room and how lovely it sounded, and she also said it was okay to go, "It's okay to go now," she said, "it's okay." At that time the patient opened her eyes and raised her head and looked at her sister in her eyes, and her sister said, "You can close your eyes and go back to sleep." She nodded, put her head down and stopped breathing; she died right there with her sister telling her that she loved her and it was okay to go, wrapped in the soothing harmonies and progression of their favorite song growing up together. So beautiful to be ushered out like that.

It seems that often people need permission to go. I have had several experiences in which a patient is lying in their deathbed and for the most part nonresponsive, they have had their family members and friends and maybe a spiritual advisor tell them it's okay and they can go, maybe God is waiting for you, they say, or your husband is waiting for you, and aren't you excited to see your kids again who have passed before you. I find that once they have been given permission, once their loved ones have conveyed that to them in an authentic way, it's not going to be too long before the patient passes.

We believe that hearing is the first sense that you get when you are in utero, and it's the very last sense that leaves before you die. So I find that it is very important for family and friends to continue to talk to their loved one, to continuously remind them that they're not alone, that they are loved, and that they have permission to go. I think more often than not that message is received. There are a lot of things that people can get hung up on when they are facing the end, so it is important to emphasize that it is okay to go, that they are loved, that everyone and everything is going to be taken care of, and whatever else may be important for them to hear before they can peacefully let go.

Sometimes people don't die the way that they want to or had anticipated. That can be hard for them and for the people around them, but that is what drives me to do my job, to make sure that all of those whom I serve have as good an experience as possible. I affirm with each of my patients that we are there for them, and if they ever need anything they can call on us and we will be there immediately. That is one reason it is so important to have an interdisciplinary team because we don't know what the patient may need but he or she will.

Sometimes people want to die alone, they don't want others to "see me like this," but I find that those are in the minority. Even knowing that people are there in spirit counts as having somebody there, they know that their loved ones are going to be with them in a spiritual sense, and that might also provide some comfort to them. Sometimes people feel guilty that they have not been with their loved one at the time of death but I tell them that they did nothing wrong, they did everything right by being there all the times that they were, offering their love and support, and it was the person's choice to die when they did.

The idea of dying alone, however, may not be what actually happens for some people. Many of my patients have mentioned that they receive visits from their loved ones who have passed on, and sometimes people say they have had a direct conversation with God. I've walked into rooms where people have stated, "I just had a conversation with God and He says it's okay to go now, it's okay to come home."

Sometimes people say that they feel the presence of their angel, of their protector, with them at all times. I've never had the experience of people receiving visitors that were unwanted or painful, it's always come as a comfort to them. About seventy percent of my patients have some kind of practicing belief system which includes a higher power or a god or angels, or loved ones who are in another world who are living and breathing, in a sense. About twenty percent of those will be forthcoming about conversations with them but it may be higher since some will not want to talk about it.

I've also walked into rooms where the patient is angry with God, they don't know why this has happened to them. Sometimes God, or the concept of a higher power is what gives people peace, but for others it is a source of stress and I have to work with that, I have to be able to meet people where they are to be able to support them. I find that if I've been referred to a patient for music therapy for spiritual support, I walk into the room representing all of their experiences with spiritual leaders. I represent the pastor they had as a child, I represent the TV evangelists, I represent all of these people, and I have to be ready to meet them on their level and support them where they are at. It's a sum total of their experiences in their spiritual community, or on the outside of their spiritual community, which leaves them at their current state of acceptance or incongruence with their spiritual beliefs and practices. Sometimes when I see people who have established a foundation on a specific religious or spiritual belief, and at the end of life that changes for them it can be very distressing.

On the other hand the opposite can happen; someone who has never believed in anything religious or spiritual can shift quite dramatically. I had a patient who never went to church, didn't really like hymns, and to use his own words thought it was a bunch of bunk. But now, facing the end of his life, he felt an undeniable presence of a spiritual figure and had an insatiable appetite for hymns and prayers and wanted it from all different denominations. He wanted to hear Buddhist prayers, he wanted to hear "The Lord's Prayer," he wanted to hear "Amazing Grace" and "How Great Thou Art," and he wanted to know about Jewish people. I'm a Jewish person so we talked a lot about that. So yes, there is absolutely a flip to the other side of the coin for some people.

There are times when a patient is referred to me who is so close to the end that it is not possible to have a conversation but we create ways to communicate anyway. I had a patient on the inpatient unit in Philadelphia, he was a fifty-five year old man who was on our service for a cancer diagnosis but he had multiple other diagnoses, as well. By the time I made my assessment visit he was no longer verbal but he was cognitively pretty sharp, I guess you could say. I was able to conduct my music therapy assessment, we came up with hand gestures for yes and no and skip. I was able to come up with a handful of songs that were particularly meaningful to him. I went in and played a few of his song, and he loved them all, he just loved them all. At one point he put out his fist for a fist bump because he really loved, "Have You Ever Seen The Rain" by Creedence Clearwater Revival. So that visit was very good.

A few days later I stopped back in his room to do a routine visit and his brothers had come into town from other states. At this time the patient was almost comatose in his bed, with occasional moaning and furrowing of his eyebrows, but most of the time he was resting pretty peacefully. His brothers asked me to play a few of the songs that he had stated were his favorites, so I played softly in the background while his brothers said their final goodbyes. They were very deep, meaningful, poetic, loving goodbyes. After about five minutes of this they got up and left the room. One of the brothers had to catch a flight back home so this really was his final goodbye.

They left, I continued playing his music softly for him in the background, and within thirty seconds of them leaving the room his heart stopped beating and he took his last breath. He died there to the tune of his favorite song. I got a nurse and they pronounced him, they called his brothers and they came right back into the room for a very tearful goodbye, appropriately so, and hugged their brother one last time before they left. I asked if they would like me to continue playing and they said yes, play him a hymn, so I played "The Lord's Prayer" and that was the final song that I played for him.

I felt the love they were emitting, they were oozing love for their brother, their baby brother. That to me was beautiful, and if anything, that might have been one of the most profound experiences for me because I am the youngest of three brothers and what I felt in that room, in addition to the bodies, was the love and the compassion, the dignity that they upheld for their brother, and the respect; that's what I felt.

As I mentioned, this man was only fifty-five years old, and I would say that nine times out of ten if I visit someone under the age of sixty they are a cancer patient. We have patients with a lot of different diagnoses, not just cancer, but respiratory pulmonary disease, kidney failure, and the majority of our older patients have some kind of dementia or Altzheimer's disease. My experience with younger people, people under the age of fifty who are not mentally ready to die, for lack of a better term, put up a fight at the end. There are those people who won't die until they are given permission to, and for younger patients who were not expecting to die so soon there is a lot of unresolved or unfinished business, maybe a lot of self-talk about not being ready to go, it's not my time. The mind affects the immune system, so if you're not totally ready to die you might prolong your life. I don't know what the quality of life is like for them at that point, if it's a life worth living or not, I can't say. Maybe for some people it is, maybe that struggling against death gives them the feeling that they've tried everything and maybe that helps get them to the place where they are ready to go.

If I do music for patients like this sometimes it helps and sometimes it doesn't. As a music therapist I am prepared to walk into a room and give a private concert, I'm prepared to walk into a room and not play any music at all, only talk, and I'm prepared to do some combination of both. For these people I find that music alone is not enough, that verbal processing is one way they might find their peace, one way they might become ready through coordinating meetings with other disciplines, maybe social work, chaplain, through coordinating a care conference with their family members and the rest of the disciplinary group who assess what's going on with the patient and what they need. Sometimes we just don't know what to provide in order to make things okay in any given moment and it will be a work in progress.

That's what hospice is all about, providing that compassion, providing that presence of someone to companionate with, someone to wade through the muck with, that's why I'm there for my people. I will sit with them through the worst of times, even if nothing more than just to offer a shoulder to cry on, or offering my stroking their forearm. There are times when the dying person feels all alone and feels that there is no hope, and sometimes it's true that they have no friends or family to be with them, and there is no hope of recovery, but there is hope of a different kind that hospice offers. You might be offered the opportunity to share your concerns, gripes, revelations, stories, wants and needs. There might be an opportunity to die in the way you always wanted to, and there is always hope that you will not die in pain. You will be shown through words and actions that you are worthy of honor and respect, and you will not be alone. This is the hospice model created by Dame Cicely Saunders (1918-2005), a nurse, social worker, physician, writer and activist who is credited with the modern-day hospice movement. She worked diligently to ease the physical, spiritual, and relationship pain of people at the end of their lives. Not everybody gets to experience this, not everybody receives hospice care, but this is what we do for the people we serve: we are there for them.

Palliative Care Overview

Application

As a medical specialty, palliative care addresses the needs of the patients and families in a whole person approach, i.e., the physical, emotional, spiritual, and relational aspects of serious illness and end-of-life care. The palliative care physician, however, does not do it alone. Palliative care is team medicine, including but not limited to other doctors, nurses, spiritual care, complementary modalities, and family involvement.

History

I don't think it is possible to give the history of palliative care as a medical specialty without looking at the history of hospice, as there is a direct lineage from one to the other.

Hospice is dedicated to helping people die in comfort. Hospice as an organization has existed in the United States since 1974, the year the first hospice was opened in Branford, Connecticut, to provide compassionate care for dying patients in their own homes. It was funded by the National Cancer Institute, but at that point it was largely a volunteer service with no medical coverage for patients. In 1979 the U.S. Congress, based upon recommendations from the U.S. Department of Health, Education, and Welfare, funded several studies to assess, among other things, costs for terminally ill hospitalized patients as compared to patients in hospice. The findings led to the approval for Medicare coverage starting in 1983, and many private insurance companies followed suit.

The person who is acknowledged as the founder of the modern-day hospice movement, Dame Cicely Saunders, MD (1918-2005), began working with dying patients in England while a nursing student, a social worker, and finally as a physician. She saw the uncontrolled pain at end of life, and the unaddressed and unmet emotional and spiritual needs. These experiences led her to her life-long mission of providing more compassionate care to the dying. This included three primary needs: to provide relief from physical pain, to help with preserving the dying person's dignity, and to help with the psychological and spiritual pain of death. These three areas are represented in hospice today as pain management, emotional and spiritual support for the patient and family, and bereavement counseling.

Requirements for licensure

To qualify as a palliative care physician one must first earn a medical degree, complete a residency in one of ten designated specialties, followed by a one-year palliative medicine fellowship accredited by the Accreditation Council for Graduate Medical Education. Although hospice as established by Dame Cicely Saunders is by definition palliative care, a person does not need to be a hospice patient to receive it. As a relatively new specialty, it was given official recognition by the American Board of Medical Specialists in 2006.

Summary

When I think about palliative care physicians, I think about the idealized view of the old country doctor; the doctor who knew his patient and the family, what he or she did for their livelihood, their economic status, their challenges, the family relationships, their religious and spiritual beliefs, their standing in the community – all of these attributes embodied by the kindly and attentive family physician.

How much of this is pure fantasy is hard to tell. Television programs such as Marcus Welby, MD, Dr. Kildare, and more contemporary medical dramas, both on prime-time television and soap operas continue to project the view of doctors who have the time, take the time, and are interested in you as a person as opposed to you as a diagnosis, a body part, or a body to be used as a teaching tool. If there are physicians who resemble the kindly old country doctor stereotype it appears that palliative care physicians, as a medical specialty, most closely fit that bill.

Telling, however, is that it appears that the more holistic the physician the less money he or she makes. On the 2016 Medscape Physician Compensation Report, palliative care physician is not listed, although it's possible that a physician may identify her or himself under another category such as oncologist. In comparing data on salary ranges for palliative care physicians from sources other than the Medscape report, palliative care physicians earn about $185,000 per year as compared to the specialties of orthopedics, at $443,000 (the highest on the Medscape list), and pediatrics at $204,000 (the lowest on the list). It seems that it takes a special kind of person to become a palliative care physician. A common sentiment among these physicians is that this is the kind of medicine they imagined practicing when they were first attracted to the profession.

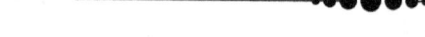

The next two interviews are with palliative care physicians, whom I have chosen to identify only as Dr. E. and Dr. K. Each has received national recognition for their leadership and commitment to creating a palliative care program in their respective clinics, hospitals, and communities, and for on-going training of medical personnel in understanding and practicing palliative care.

I have chosen to identify them by an initial only because they spoke to me about deeply personal issues which, in my experience, is rare for a doctor to do. As medical professionals they may or may not wish to share these details with the general public; I will leave that up to them. I appreciate their openness with me as it provides a look into palliative medicine, and may give some insight into why a physician would choose to go for further training to become a specialist in this field, dedicated to relieving the suffering of those with terminal illnesses.

Dr. E.
Palliative Care Physician

Introduction

Dr. E. works in a West Coast cancer center with most of his patients seen in clinic as an outpatient, with a few inpatients.

Interview

Our palliative care clinic has only been open since 2008 and I would say probably eighty percent plus of the patients I take care of eventually enroll and die in hospice care; that's a common thing. The longer that I practice the more chronically ill patients are in my practice, so I have a small cohort of those, as well. Everybody dies, but not immediately.

Once a patient is enrolled in hospice, my role is largely determined by which hospice they are receiving services from. There are probably a dozen hospices in this area and I don't believe there is one that is clearly better than the others, nor do I believe that there is one that patients need to avoid; they all have their different strengths and limitations. For the most part I've been pretty uniformly impressed by the dedication and caring of the people who are involved. Most of the difficulties arise over resources and allocations of resources; will they pay for this or that, and that's really not the hospice's fault, that's the way US healthcare is structured.

When I talk to a patient about hospice care, I usually think about it in terms of whether or not they are getting treatments that are going to be a potential barrier to hospice. There are some treatments that are simply too expensive for hospices to afford, and at other times there are treatments that a patient may want that a hospice may or may not approve. For example, there are some patients who want to receive intravenous fluids and some hospices really discourage that, some hospices are willing to support it for a limited time, and some hospices are pretty open to doing it. I've had some patients who are on intravenous pain pumps and some of the hospices are quite okay with those and others are not.

Some patients have limitations on which hospice they can use, either geographically or based on their insurance. I mostly encourage them to invite the hospice out and meet them and talk with them. Then they have the option of deciding to enroll or not after they hear how it works. If they have treatments that I am concerned that there may be problems for the hospice to support, then I ask them to communicate directly with the hospice and see what they say.

I rarely make home visits once hospice is going in; I find that is sufficient. It's not for lack of wanting to, I'd love visiting patients in their homes, it's my favorite thing to do, but I've reached the point in my career where there's just not time in my life and really, nobody wants to pay how much it would cost for me to go and visit all of my patients at home. There's no entity that's interested in funding that, it would be pretty expensive.

I do make some home visits, but usually it's more to people who are really struggling before they make a decision to enroll in hospice. Once they're enrolled in hospice the most common role that I play is I'm there sort of as their attending doctor, but sometimes I won't play any role at all. Those are the two most common roles: no role or as their attending physician in hospice.

Now days there are hospice doctors and hospices have medical directors. Some of the hospices really take over, and there are a lot of physicians who don't think they know how, or don't prioritize, or don't feel like they have the time to be the attending physician for their hospice patients. There is also the issue of whether or not they will be reimbursed, so a lot of hospices employ their own directors and those doctors generally take over. Other hospices really work to keep the patient's doctor involved as sort of the center, at least where all of the orders are coming from, and things like that. Different hospices have different levels of medical director involvement, although the trend is for more, over time, now that it is a recognized specialty.

Why did I go into palliative care? To begin with, the decision to become a doctor was really just a suggestion from my mother, I would credit her with it. She thought it was a good career, and I remember her saying that it's such a broad field that once you go into it there are still lots of different directions you can go. Since I wasn't sure what I was good at, or what I wanted, that notion of still having a lot of options appealed to me. If I'm completely honest about why I chose palliative care, the answer changes over time, how I understand why I decided to do it changes over time, but the closest I can come to it is that it comes from the same place as a parent's love for their child.

The point in my life where I decided to go into palliative care followed, maybe a year after my wife and I tried to have a baby and had a miscarriage. After that I actually became depressed, and as I was coming out of the depression I got this idea that I would go do a palliative care fellowship. I really didn't understand the link between the two, or if there was one, until years later when I went to a workshop with Rachael Naomi Remen, M.D. author of *Kitchen Table Wisdom*, (1994). She said, "Bring something with you, bring an object with you that symbolizes why you do what you do, the work that you do." And she said, "If you don't know, don't think about it too hard, just grab the first thing that comes to mind and bring it, and we'll talk about it when you get here."

So I grabbed my object and showed up at the workshop, and then we did this little exercise where we sat around in small groups and we talked about our object. I was absolutely thunderstruck when it was my turn, I couldn't speak. I don't know how long I sat there trying to speak and not being able to say anything, but I would guess it was close to ten minutes of just, I just couldn't talk. That's a long time for a small group of people to sit there. Everybody was like, "Holy crap, what's going to happen?"

I don't even remember what I said after that, but the object that

I brought was Jizo Bodhisattva, which is a little statue of a deity that symbolizes the protector of children. So I think the reason I do what I do is the motivation that comes from the same place that a parent's love for his or her child comes from.

Part of my work is to relieve suffering, and I would say, also, that I'm looking to create benefit and to identify and help people move in ways that are beneficial. What that exactly looks like depends on what is beneficial for them. I depend on the patient to help me understand what is quality of life, what is beneficial for him or her, because it's different for everybody, and it's often a moving target. I'm an expert in palliative care but I can't be an expert in what is quality of life for them, so I really try to encourage people to talk, what is most important to them, what they're afraid of, what they're hoping for, what they are wishing for, and as they talk I do often get ideas, or suggestions come up of ways to proceed that might be beneficial. We are looking at the whole person, so it may very well include physical, emotional, mental, and spiritual aspects of who they are.

I've come to realize that there is not a lot of death in dying, it's really not evident to me. Some people are clearly dying, but that's such a short time. What's much more evident is that even people who are terminally ill and expected to die, the challenge is, well, how do you live? That's what they're doing, they're not dying, they're really living, or trying to figure out how to. So there is very little dying or death, they're alive and living, and there's dead, so the death and dying piece is really just a little microscopic piece in there.

In the search for how to live, many of my patients utilize complementary and alternative treatments. I don't do them myself, but since I am based in a cancer center, and cancer patients are really proactive and engaged in their treatment options, they discuss what they are doing with me. I think that often what they're looking for within traditional health care, they're looking for doctors who can support what they're doing, or engage with them. A lot of doctors will say, "Well, I don't really know much about that," the patient will try to talk about it and the physician is like, "Well, it's probably okay." The way that I frame it for people is that my view of alternative and complementary treatments, if you want to call them that, is that their orientation is that they're trying to activate the body's intrinsic intent to heal, trying to align yourself with that capacity and strengthen and activate it.

My view is what will do that for an individual is very personal. Often we will get family members who are very enthusiastic about them and really want their family member to try it, but the patient is really not that excited about it. I tell the family, "If the patient hears about it and says, 'that makes sense to me, I would like to try it,' " and it's not too toxic or too expensive, then I encourage them to try it and pay attention to the results. Are they getting better? Are they feeling better? If they are, then they should continue, and if they try it and that's not the case, then they can move on. So I sort of encourage them to use the empirical approach because, first of all, what patients are often seeking is a way they can really engage, they want to be involved in getting better. Some of the treatments that we give to people, it seems that stuff is being done to you and you're in more of a passive position, and this gives them the opportunity to take a more active role. Many of them find that energizing and activating, and I really want to support that.

Like any treatment, results will vary, but usually the level of toxicity of alternative and complementary treatments is pretty low. I tell patients that one of the prerequisites of this is that you really need to think, really believe that it is going to help you, and then when you do it you need to have that sense that it is benefitting you. If you don't have that sense then you probably ought not to continue. But patients ask me, "Well, isn't that like the placebo effect?" and I say, "What do you think the placebo effect is? It's the body's intrinsic capacity to heal, that's exactly what it is, so don't discount it: it's the basis for all healing, nothing to turn your nose up at." If you've been healed before then you know the value.

Some patients consult with me about the value of continuing an alternative or complementary treatment, sometimes because they don't want to continue it and are hesitant to tell a family member, sometimes they need permission to stop, and sometimes they just need more information. I remember one patient who was taking painful injections and was willing to continue if there was evidence that it was helping, but the treatment had not stopped the progression or made it better. Could you say it was progressing slower because of the treatment? We really couldn't answer that question, sometimes you just don't know.

I don't know anything about Healing Touch or Therapeutic Touch or Reiki in any kind of expert fashion. I think that, well, what I think is that over time and with experience, people whose intention it is to foster healing or help people feel better become the medicine themselves, they become a therapeutic intervention themselves. How exactly one does that, I think, depends upon the individual and how they connect. My intervention is just to listen to people. It would probably be more potent if I used some type of touch or something like that, but I find it is sufficient for me to really listen.

I do a practice that Rachael Remen gave me called *Generous Listening.* That's sort of my principle practice or way of relating to patients. I will read what she said from this paper that I carry with me; her language is exquisite.

> *When we listen we're usually thinking. We may be deciding if we like or dislike what is being said, if we agree with it or not, if we believe it or not. We may be listening competitively, we may be listening with an agenda. As health professionals we are trained to listen for what is wrong and are concerned with whether or not we know how to fix it. In listening generously we do not do any of this; we just listen in silence, not to analyze, or even to understand. We're listening simply to know what is true for another person at this time. When we do this, we often enable someone to recognize what is true for them, for the first time.*

This is sometimes true but you don't always know about it. But I think that the other thing that happens, in my experience of doing the practice since 2007, is that it changes the quality of the way that you listen to people and with time, as I put it before, you sort of become the medicine.

People don't always talk to me about their dying and death but they do sometimes. I think that some people are worried about dying, about the process itself, that's what they're worried about, they're worried about what's going to happen, so sure, people talk about that sometimes. I ask them, "What are you most worried about?" and that comes up fairly frequently. The other practice that I do, although it's not something I do consciously, is called *giving the gift of no fear*, a concept taught by the author and Zen teacher, Joan Halifax. Since I'm not the one whose death we're talking about, and also because I have talked to a lot of people about this, I tend not to get alarmed by their conversation and I can have a fairly benign, matter-of-fact conversation about dying and what will happen in a way that I think can be therapeutic for some people.

I had a patient who was obsessed about talking to everybody about her dying, so she would engage everybody in conversation, you couldn't come within her radius without her wanting to talk about it. Because she had her cancer for about eight years she became very, very good about talking about it and engaging people, sometimes funny, sometimes with humor, she had all kinds of different ways of doing it. By the time I met her she was really good about talking about it and she didn't have to use all of her tricks with me. I had the unique privilege of talking to her on the last day of her life and I was thanking her: I told her it was sort of a relief to talk to somebody who isn't afraid of dying. She kind of laughed and said, "But Doctor, I'm still afraid of dying, I'm just not afraid to talk about it." I realized that was really true, she was not afraid to talk about it. When the time actually came, she turned out not to be particularly afraid of death, either. She may have thought she was afraid of it, but when it was actually happening she was not. But I thought that was interesting, somebody who you think is not afraid of it because they talk about it all the time can still be afraid of it: there's a difference between the actual event and the talking about it.

Being able to talk openly about dying and death is some of the value that people in palliative care can bring, and do bring: it's such an unusual gift or quality that I think it's quite exquisite. At the same time it's not something that people are necessarily looking for. It's been an aspect of palliative care that is not put out in front because we want people not to be afraid or put off by the death-i-ness of the profession.

••••●●●••

I'm not with a person at the time of their death very often. One reason is that most of them die in their homes, and if they die in the hospital I will usually have done my piece in the patient care and then I need to move to the next thing. There are stories of the dying person seeing deceased loved ones and talking to people that nobody else can see, but in my personal experience most of those stories come from hospice care and are extremely rare in the hospital. Many of the patients that I'm dealing with are in the hospital, and in the hospital there is very, very low tolerance for people being awake and dying. If you die in the hospital you are almost invariably sedated, either because you are uncomfortable or the people around you are uncomfortable. The chance that nobody is uncomfortable, and nobody gets sedated in that situation, it almost never happens.

I try to help people not die in the hospital because I think the potential for healing and being awake is just greater at home, but it's not always possible. Some people really do need to die in the hospital, and some families are just not equipped to deal with them dying at home. However, I think it's very, very human for people to not want to die in the hospital where everybody is scared, they're all scared of dying, it's a place that is dedicated to not dying, it's not a place that has a wide comfort zone and acceptance for dying. And of course the families want the patient to be comfortable, and they're sitting there and they're anxious, so if anything happens they ask for something to treat the patient so we do. We err on the side of comfort, and in the hospital we have all kinds of medications we can give them, it's very easy to give them, and we can give them by any route, whether they can swallow or not.

Regardless of what is happening, I try not to look at the circumstances of somebody's dying and just see all the things that are wrong with it, I notice those things, but I also try to see what else is there and invariably it's never all good or all bad. Some of the most anxious and difficult families also have a great deal of love and strength and courage, so I try to draw attention to that. Some patients get agitated and out of control at the end of their lives and that's really hard to watch, but at the same time you see families and health professionals really heroically trying to make the situation better. I wish it wasn't that way, but when it actually happens I find plenty of good to go with the bad, I guess is the best way to put it.

That extreme agitation at the end, that's really the hardest thing. We see it a lot in younger men, especially people who are physically strong. It's often the most challenging situation that we not infrequently encounter in end-of-life care, and it's the reason we sedate people, for sure. For others at the end, they may become delirious and they just don't have the energy or the strength to be very agitated.

Being in the presence of great suffering is definitely a real challenge, a hard part, probably the hardest part of my job, and remaining open in that situation and consistently showing up, especially when it's protracted over a long period of time. We've had patients who have been in and out of that extremely agitated state over a significant length of time. We had a patient like that who was in the hospital for over a year. The only person who was able to remain engaged over the entire year was the nurse on our team, she managed to stay connected in some way with the patient. Our chaplain tried, but he got fired by the patient at some point so he couldn't go back. He probably would have hung in there if he had been allowed to.

When I was a young doctor Rachael Remen was at Harvard to introduce her book and a course she was teaching. After the presentation I went to get my book signed and she asked me what I did. I said I was a palliative care fellow and she said, "Isn't that wonderful." I didn't say anything, and she said "Isn't it?" I said, "Well, it's just really difficult working with people who are suffering and dying all the time," and without missing a beat she just looked at me and said, "Well, it's only difficult if you think the world is broken and it's your job to fix it."

So now here is the conundrum: How am I supposed to experience the world in which nothing is broken and it's not my job to fix it, yet in my chosen profession I see suffering all the time and my intention is to relieve suffering? Maybe both things are true. Ultimately, what is healing is presence. If you are present in the presence of suffering it's difficult but not degrading, and all of the things that are stressful, if they happen in the context of you being present, they really are pretty manageable. It's when I kind of get caught outside of that, when all of a sudden I realize that my mind has gone somewhere else, that is challenging; there's an infinite number of invitations to not be present.

My experience is that the work is emotionally demanding, and some of the stories are distressing, and the suffering is often very intense and very real. Bad things happen to people that I care about, so within that I experience all kinds of emotional things and ideas and whatnot, but probably the most common experience is one of grief. There is a Zen story about a guy who is being installed at a monastery and part of the ceremony was taking questions from the audience. Somebody asked him the question, "So, how do we care for others?" And the new Abbott responded, "What others? Care for yourself." So the questioner said, "Alright, then, how do we care for ourselves?" And the Abbott said, "Care for others."

In order to continue to work in the field I find that I have to do many things to take care of myself: I exercise, I meditate, I am deeply involved in my faith community, and I have colleagues that I share this experience with, so I spend a tremendous amount of time with self-care. If you had told me when I was starting out that I would have to spend the amount of hours that I do on self-care I probably would have said, "Oh, well, I better find a different profession."

So it literally is, "How do you take care of others? You take care of yourself." If I didn't take care of others I wouldn't take care of myself the way that I do, so it seems like a little Zen koan, but actually, for me, it's very pragmatic and literally true. I would say all of these things are a lot of the best things that I do, so I'm actually blessed to have a job that forces me to do them because I probably wouldn't do them if I had an easier job.

The worst part of my job is also the best part. There's a lot of joy in palliative and end-of-life care; it has an exquisite quality to it because of the circumstances it occurs in. Some of it is joy when people are doing well, sometimes good things go well and you're like "Yeah," delighted! We see people in these difficult circumstances and more often than not you find something to admire about them; their goodness kind of activates your goodness. I would say that joy is really there, it's right there next to all the other stuff, but it's really there. Few people would say that but that's just because they really don't know what it is like to be fully present with your life and with your experiences in the moment, seeing and feeling the love; there can be joy in that.

One of the things that people who work in my field may come to learn is that grief is not bad, it doesn't harm you. If it did, then we'd have the worst job in the world and nobody would want to do it, for good reason, but it's actually not harmful. It can be harmful, but only if you really struggle against it, I think. So if you can allow it to work on you then it does its work and something comes next.

One of the things that has changed for me as I have worked in this field is my ability to abide in the mystery in death, the mystery of what happens after you die. I think increasingly I'm able to tolerate not knowing the answer to that, just being with the question and the mystery. I think if you can find a way to have an honest and heartfelt conversation about death with somebody that you trust, that is beneficial; it makes talking about it less scary, it makes thinking about it less scary. It doesn't take the fear away completely because I think we are programmed to be afraid of dying, but that fear is one of the main drivers to appreciating and feeling grateful for our lives. So I don't think that one needs to get rid of that fear, but if you can find the courage to talk about it, I think that's beneficial.

Dr. K.
Bachelor of Science, Biochemistry
MD
Medical Director of Palliative Care

Introduction

Dr. K. is a pioneer in the field of palliative medicine, starting the first program of its kind in a large Western state hospital. He cites the year 2000 as the year he first identified as a palliative care specialist, but it was not until 2006 that hospice and palliative medicine was officially recognized by the American Board of Medical Specialties. He sees patients in the hospital and in hospice care and shares stories of visits to patients in their homes.

Interview

My mother's death was brutal, just brutal, but there were many gifts in it for me: it's what led me to my true calling as a palliative care physician.

I had graduated from high school and had no plans on going to college, so I went across the country, started out in California, and I was in a commune for a brief period of time. Coming back on a Greyhound bus, somewhere around the middle of the country I decided that I had to figure out what I was going to do with my life. I thought, well, why not be a doctor? I had certain gifts, I was smart enough, so I had chosen to be a doctor before I had any experience, any personal experience or any end-of-life experience. I enrolled in a junior college, transferred to a university, and shortly after I transferred to UC Davis, at the end of my second year my mother had a stroke.

The stroke actually turned out to be due to lung cancer. This was in 1980, so at that time the treatments were much harsher than they are now and communication was much different than it is now. She had a complete pneumonectomy, removal of the entire lung, she had radiation, she had chemotherapy, and she lived for twenty-one months after her diagnosis. She was forty-eight when she was diagnosed and she died at forty-nine. She was a smoker, smoked Pall Malls, unfiltered, and her treatment and death were brutal, tremendously brutal.

Between my third and fourth year of college I took the year off. I lived with my folks and worked, and I was with my mother pretty much every day. I think I was her main source of strength during that time, my father and myself, but I had more time with her than he did; I was with her a lot more. Having that year, or most of the year with her, caring for her and watching her die slowly, watching the loss of this rich, robust, luscious person, and how the treatment more than the disease took pieces away from her bit by bit was such an emotionally intense experience for me.

As difficult as my mother's death was for me, there were also many gifts as a result. The closeness, the affection and love that we had for each other, it came to the forefront and it was very strong. She had been raised in a very conventional family, had a very conventional husband, and she had always longed, I think, to break free of that mold but had trouble doing it, so in many respects her illness gave her a little bit more freedom in how she thought and acted. She read Elizabeth Kubler-Ross' book, *On Death and Dying*, and she went to a workshop or two. For her I think it was very spiritually enriching to have to be in the moment faced with her mortality, and for me it was just a very emotionally intense experience.

I visited my mom in the hospital the evening before she died, and I just remember her being irritable and cranky and phobic and restless, and I thought "This isn't what it is supposed to be like." When she died I wept for three days, and then I started to study for the medical college admission test. I read text books, notes, this and that, and scored very high on the test. Then, after the test, I wouldn't say I fell apart, that wasn't it at all, but the enormity of what had happened, and the loss, none of which sounds like much of a gift, but there were a number of gifts, one of which was the morning she died.

I remember getting the call, my sister and my father got the call and woke us all up, just this spiritually desolate experience, this feeling of bleakness. But a few hours later as I am going for a walk, which is the way I coped throughout her illness, going on long, long walks and singing as I went along, I'm walking through the mist at the base of the foothills and all of a sudden my mother is everywhere, just the essence of who she was, was everywhere. There were no more visitations from her after that.

The years went by and her illness and death certainly colored my medical school experience in that I was unique, and I would ask medical school students for years afterwards, "How many of you have had a first-degree family member die?" There might be one out of ten, and of those, "How many of you were there for the last months of life?" maybe one in a hundred had been. So it was a unique experience for me as compared to the people that I worked with and went to school with.

I had always wanted to do hospice care but for some reason I never thought it was possible, that you had to be somebody really special to do that. My experience as a medical director of a nursing home, then a medical director for hospice beginning in the mid 90s, showed me how little priority older people were given, with missed diagnoses, doctors just going through the motions, and it was brutal, just like my mother's treatment was brutal. I started to diagnose Parkinson's disease that hadn't been treated, started allowing people to die, started taking feeding tubes out: it was beautiful, I loved working at the nursing home.

At that time there were very few hospice programs in my town and for the most part they were run by oncologists. The joke in the medical profession about hospice in those days was that the hospice medical director had three jobs: show up, shut up, and sign things, meaning that he or she was just a figurehead. But I didn't know how to be a hospice doctor, so I showed up, asked questions, I made suggestions, I argued with my staff, and I went out and saw patients. I was reading an awful lot, a voracious reader, trying to figure out how to do this.

I remember one of my early experiences when the nurses were talking about going to see a patient and I said, "Let's go see him." This was a man with metastatic prostate cancer who was relatively healthy other than cancer and metastises, and he was going to have a spinal cord compression if we didn't do anything. With a cord compression he would have been paralyzed, so for the last six months of his life he would have been unable to walk, he would have been incontinent, and to me that didn't seem like good care, it didn't seem like good end-of-life care. So I told him he should revoke hospice, get radiation, and then he should get back on hospice.

Now, the ironic thing was that his oncologists were both medical directors of hospices and here I am kicking him off of our hospice, sending him back to the oncologists. As we were leaving his house the nurse said to me, "I've never had a doctor be there with me before." It just struck me. So, not knowing how things were done I did what I thought should be done and it led to some very wonderful experiences, tremendously wonderful experiences caring for people.

He got radiation, he came back on hospice, and he lived several months. I think he did well with some quality of life until at the very end he struggled, he needed a lot of medicine and was agitated, which surprised me. But years later this woman stops me as I was walking out of the hospital, stops me, says hello, and it was his daughter. He lived at home and it was much easier for the family to have him there. I don't know all that happened, but changing the trajectory from a bad to a good death changes things for the patient, the family, and for friends.

That was in the late 90s, and about the same time we started an HIV clinic. Part of the reason that I started that was because AIDS was a new disease while I was in medical school so I knew as much about it as anybody in town, and it was end-of-life care for people my own age. A few months afterwards was when all the breakthroughs happened with highly active therapy and instead of being end-of-life care it became chronic disease management.

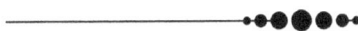

The year 2000 is when I mark the beginning of my true career as a specialist in palliative care. It's here that I think my mother's gift really became evident and that was a need, a passion, with a lot of counter transference at first, to do a good job. Her death had been something to dread, the experience with my mother was terrible, and I wanted to make it different for other people.

The first time I cared for a 50-year-old woman with lung cancer I wasn't aware of how much my mother's death was influencing my professional opinions. I was angry at the oncologist for giving up on this woman with advanced metastatic lung cancer, who had metastases in her spine and in her neck, she had an unstable neck, and she died a week after I saw her, if that. I was thinking, "The oncologist should have a neurosurgeon stabilize her spine so her performance status would improve so she could get chemotherapy." I mean, talk about counter transference, and when she died I realized "this is kind of nuts," what I was thinking.

So with the next lung cancer woman who was 50 years old it was different, and the one after that was even more different. I asked my students, "What's the difference between counter transference and wisdom?" because they're both related to past experience. I think the difference is insight. The gift of my mother is that I would go out on a limb and I had company going out on a limb, I wasn't afraid to go out on a limb, and that's necessary to introduce palliative care to this community in the hospital setting.

As I took care of a series of fifty-year-old women, the last one was my mother in so many respects. I saw her in the hospital one weekend and I looked at her and said, "Oh my, it doesn't have to be like this, it doesn't have to be so terrible." The woman, who didn't speak English, had an interpreter with her and as I left the room after telling them that I would intervene and make things better the interpreter was crying, the family was crying, and the nursing case manager was crying, but I wasn't crying. Treatment at a certain stage can be likened to torture, with very little benefit. Sometimes it's hard to know what to do but in this case I knew, and I felt that I had really done something.

She lived in a small rural town and a week later I went to see her. I walked into this old farmhouse and she came out with such pride. There was a picture on her piano, this rich hair, luscious, just full of life. I looked at her and asked, "Is that you?" and she smiled and nodded. So much like my mother, who played piano, too. I came home from that visit, once again grieving my mother's death, but something had shifted and I was able to put it to rest. It was the right thing to do, to grow up and move on, but it didn't make going out on a limb easier, it made it lonelier.

———————————•◦●◦●◦•———————————

First and foremost when I take care of patients is to make a connection with them. I wouldn't say that I have stock phrases that I use, but tools that may be applicable. One of them is when I'm reading the patient's chart and I watch people go in and out and in and out of the room, and I walk in and here is this person who's demoralized and despondent and I'll ask, "Never have you had so much attention, right?" And they'll say, "Yeah." "And never have you felt more alone." And they say, "No."

When I am asked to do a consult I will review the charts, get a sense of what's going on medically, then show up with sometimes no idea of how I am going to approach something, but I don't need to have an idea, I really just need to show up. Sometimes I'll be eloquent in introducing myself, other times I muddle through, and sometimes it's the muddling that is disarming so that I can make that connection. Before I go into the room I have to really consider, "Well, what's my intention? What is my motivation, what do I want to do? Do I want to convince this person to change their code status, do I want to convince this family to take the person off the ventilator, or they shouldn't have any more chemotherapy?" If that's my motivation then I need to recognize it and let go of it and to consider, "What is my real motivation?" which is the easing of suffering, then engage the person, genuinely.

I'm a lot more constrained now than I was when I first started in palliative care because nobody knew what palliative care was -- external constraints, I mean, not personal or internal. Now we have metrics that need to be attended to, expectations for how we practice. I'll give you an example.

Our medical record notes have to follow a template. Before, I would dictate or write a note and it would speak to what was going on versus with electronic medical records there are all these little fields that need to be filled out, many of which are pre-populated, which include extraneous information that results in the message getting completely lost. With every patient I am required to ask certain questions even though they may not be pertinent or even appropriate to what is going on. For example, one that I have trouble with is under family history, which is a weird place for it to be, we have to ask the question, "Are you at peace?" Well, it's a good question unless you *have* to ask it, and if you *have* to ask it it's just by rote rather than it being a question that can create a genuine connection.

If you are suffering you are not at peace. One aspect of suffering that I incorporate with some patients is the idea that suffering is a threat to the integrity of the person, to the view of who they are, their self-concept. Let me give you an example.

I had a patient whose profession was communication, making videos and audios. He wasn't an actor but that's what he did. He developed chronic lymphocytic leukemia and was given a medication that put him into remission but has an infrequent side effect of causing something called progressive multi-focal encephalopathy (PML) which is a condition very similar to Huntington's chorea. The thing with Huntington's chorea, though, is that it takes years and years to develop, whereas with PML it's like Huntington's chorea squeezed into about three months. So here was this man in his late 50s, early 60s, who went from working to being incontinent, not able to swallow, drooling, unable to speak clearly, who had been told of a treatment that had been given to a handful of patients.

I drive out to his home to see him because I was asked to help counsel him on what's the right thing to do. I have no idea what's the right thing. I do know that the treatment is not covered by insurance, some people who have received it have stabilized and one has improved, it would cost somewhere on the order of $100,000.00, and he would have to go out of town for the treatment.

It's summer, and when I got out of the car I could hear lawnmowers, kids playing baseball, I knock on the door and go in, and here's this guy with a stained tank top, just sitting there, drooling. I go over, stoop right beside him and I say, "Who are you?" I had no plans of doing that, kind of a weird thing to do, and he answers in a very garbled manner, "I'm a regular guy." And I said, "A regular, guy." "Yeah." "And regular guys don't drool, they don't wear diapers, do they?" "No." I asked, "Is the hardest thing about this is that you have lost who you think you are?" "That's it, exactly."

So I said, "Who are you, really? You're the guy who does the video stuff, yeah, who else are you?" So we start working through who he was. He was a husband, a breadwinner. So I said, "Yeah, those are your roles: who else are you?" He looked at me and I asked, "Do you like the sound of birds singing?" And he said, "Yeah." "So you're someone who likes listening to the birds sing. Do you like the feel of wind on your face?" He says, "Yes." So as we talked about who he was, there's this narrow part of him that was his professional role, so I said, "You have a choice here of taking this treatment, rolling the die, and there's a chance you'll recover part way, unlikely you'll recover all the way, there's a chance you'll stay like this, and there's a chance you'll die. What is certain is that you'll spend a hundred thousand dollars and you'll be out of town and the whole focus will be on the disease. You won't have an open window in the hospital where you'll hear birds singing, you won't feel the breeze on your face, but you can have a lot more certainty with the other choice. If you choose to stay here you can be certain that you can have your window open, and you can know that much of who you are as a person is still valid. How would it be to die, not thinking that you gave up on your chance, but to know you seized the opportunity to make sure someone you love is better off?" So right then and there he chose hospice. But when I went to see him a couple of weeks later he's in this room, it's overheated, the window is closed, and I say, "Oh no, no, no, this is not who he is; he's not the person who lays and suffers in a room." We had to change that.

My job in this case was to ask questions, give information, and support the final decision. In other cases where I am the attending physician rather than just a consultant, there are times I have to set limits and say what I will and will not do. I had a man who was dying, his skin was falling off, he was awake and conscious and would scream, or try to scream but couldn't because he had a ventilator, when he had his dressings changed. I want to know "Why are we doing this?" A couple of days prior we had talked to his wife about changing him to a no resuscitation order, and then she wanted to change it back to full code. I said, "We're not going to do that." And she said, "Are you allowed to not do what I tell you?" And I said, "yes, we are; we're not required to perform ritual torture, we're not going to do it. You can find somebody else who will, but not me."

That's not how I would ordinarily deal with something, but in this case I had an obligation to protect this man and the ability to do so, but if I merely set up an adversarial relationship I don't do anything, I don't help anyone. So a lot of it is to try to understand who these people are and what it is that drives them, what is it that would drive them to harm someone whom they love? The skill sometimes is in finding the right time and the right manner to communicate with them. You invite them into dialogue. A lot of time family has been put in a position where they feel they have to dig in their heels to maintain or find some sense of control. If I can approach them, believing, if only in the moment that these people really want to do the right thing, or they are so hurt and frightened they have no choice, then I can work with them, and it's as much my frame of reference as it is theirs. We can talk about the facts of the case and cycle around with those, what can or can't be done, for example, but underlying it all is an emotional dynamic that's driving the process, and that process will continue until that emotional dynamic is recognized and addressed. Asking a question such as "Are you afraid?" brings the conversation to something that is very real to them.

I don't often use the term "good death" because it seems presumptuous somehow. I'm not sick, so if I am talking to a family or a patient I rarely use that term. I'll say it a little differently, I'll say, "You know, there's a myth that this has to be terrible, it doesn't have to be terrible, it can be wonderful, it can be a beautiful experience for everybody. Sad, yes, but not bad." I've said that many times.

As a palliative care physician I have the luxury of being able to spend time with my patients. On a busy day I may see seven or eight patients, maybe be able to spend two hours with somebody. Just when the palliative care department was being established at my hospital there were two heart patients whose conditions were almost identical, and the difference in their treatment is a good example of standard medical care as compared to palliative care.

The first patient was a woman who had had a cardiac arrest, she had no likelihood of any decent functional outcome, and three weeks later she's still on the ventilator, receiving standard medical care, and every day the physician writes a note, orders labs, changes this thing or that thing, and doesn't spend any time with the family. She lived like this for three weeks, and over that time an awful lot of time, effort, and money went into caring for this person.

A couple of months later another person is admitted to the hospital who is almost identical to the first patient, and since we were a new service and I didn't have other patients yet I was able, over the course of at least six hours, to spend time with the family from the time they came into the ER to the time of death, so six hours versus twenty-one days. It seems like a lot of time, but if you think of it more in a longitudinal perspective it's almost always a very efficient use of time.

The problem is that we're not paid, hospitals aren't paid, to necessarily do what's best for the patient; we're paid to see people and document a certain way to do procedures. Hospitals usually support palliative care even though on paper they lose money, but in actuality they save money. For every patient that I see the hospital is going to save somewhere between two thousand and ten thousand dollars. Saving the hospital money is not my intention, it's a consequence of doing the right thing, of finding what is really good quality care, and quality care is less expensive over the long run. Our length of stays are not shorter, they're longer probably, but they're also cheaper because we start cutting back a lot of the things the patient doesn't want that are expensive and that don't make sense. Some of it is really simple. If I have a stable patient who needs to be woken up every four hours for vitals, and they're also having to wear wires, and there's noise in the hospital, and they're uncomfortable, they don't get any sleep, they stay in the hospital longer. I can do something as simple as "No, do not awaken for vitals," and the patient sleeps better. If I can control their pain better they sleep better, they get better sooner, and it's cheaper.

It used to be that if we got a patient out of the hospital sooner we would make more money; it's not that we save money, we make money. In a medical system where neutropenic fevers, fevers caused by chemotherapy and other cancer treatments, and surgical complications are profitable, it creates a perverted set of considerations for hospital administrators and others in the system. For some conditions now, if a patient has to be readmitted to a hospital within thirty days after discharge for the same condition they were originally hospitalized for, the hospital is not paid for either the first or the second hospitalization.

Sometimes we release a patient too soon because we don't pay attention to those things that are going to make a difference to them coming back. From a public health model paying attention to those things that would cause readmission and providing palliative care makes a lot of sense, but from a corporate model that isn't necessarily the case although that is changing, and changing rapidly.

Some years ago I heard a lecture about ethical concerns related to palliative sedation from the perspective of what actually happens to various aspects of a person on a more spiritual level when they die, and that sense of home-coming in the very last minutes for some people. A question from the audience was about the difference between a palliativist as compared to a palliative care specialist, and the presenter said it is the words "special care." It made me think about hospice and palliative care. Hospice is not all about evidence-based outcomes, it's not all about medicine, it is really about love. For most of the people who work in hospice it really is a labor of love. As hospice changes and becomes more accessible I see changes both good and bad: accessibility is positive, but if it becomes just medicine it loses something.

The best part of my job is making a connection with a person and knowing it made a difference for them, that they lived well in their last hours, days, weeks, months, years; that's the best part, to know that that happened. Sometimes it happens in front of me, sometimes it's more of a knowledge or awareness, but it's not a witnessing. It doesn't matter.

The worst part is when I have a sense of futility, and I feel that I really don't have any skills as a healer, I'm going through the motions, and I'm waiting until I can retire because I'm exhausted and burned out. I don't want to retire, I want to enjoy my work, but if I can't enjoy my work then that's when I want to retire. The other worst part is when I walk into the room and I feel empty and I have nothing to give the person and I feel like a fool; I don't have the answers to any of their questions and it's just awkward and uncomfortable. That happens from time to time.

Eric Cassell, MD, talks about the universal components of human suffering, one of which is isolation loneliness, so you have somebody who is trying to help them with medication and this and that versus *being* with them. So what I see of Healing Touch is that it allows nurses and others to care for a patient rather than just doing tasks. I do recognize that I have a limited set of tools as a doctor. I can do more and more over time, and my colleagues can do more and more to deal with the body, but in terms of dealing with the person or the planet or the community or a family, the tools are limited but still very important. I think one of the best palliative care doctors is a good obstetrician who prevents years of suffering from cerebral palsy. That is care that helps the community, the family, and the person; it's very important.

I was with a dying man last night, and as with all the thousands of people I have cared for I really wanted to help him and it was really hard. He would be agitated, he would be restless, and he would refuse medication. So I ended up under-medicating him even though he was in terrible, terrible, terrible body pain: I felt helpless. It would have been wonderful to have some integrative care, a hospice volunteer or hospice nurse, a complementary medicine component, because the care wasn't integrated, it was compartmentalized. I recognize the worth of alternative and complementary modalities but I have no skill in them so I was not able to offer them to my dying patient.

As with many of the alternative therapies I'm ignorant. It's not that

I discount them but I don't know, truly, what they are. I have a sense of what Healing Touch is, of meridians and energy flows and so forth, and, I would say, a perception of a world view that I can understand in an abstract sense, but it's not the paradigm under which I have studied and learned to practice, so there's a fair amount of, I wouldn't say willful ignorance, but ignorance. One of my questions about Healing Touch is how much of it is the moving of energy, the perception of energy, and how much of it is presence and intuition and being with a person and they feeling that they are important enough for somebody to spend time with them. Really, maybe they're not doing anything that the person can see, but they're spending time.

I think as physicians we are specialists in the body and to an extent the psyche, and I think Healing Touch deals with energy and life force and things such as love, which are not necessarily acceptable words in science and medicine. The paradigm of hospitals is not based on healing, and if it is based on healing it's a very mechanistic paradigm; there is no room in that paradigm for anything that is not material. Some hospital administrations will tolerate it, not all, and very few will support it because they don't see the value. Asking most hospital administrators, medical directors, and probably a lot of nursing leaders to consider incorporating energy-based healing methods into standard care is difficult because they are most likely going to view it as voodoo. We don't even touch on the power of the mind in medical school, although they do a bit better job of it in specialty pain management clinics.

What do I want to say about death? It's easy, anybody can do it. I had a dream not long ago and in the dream somebody asked, "What is it like to die?" I usually don't remember dreams, and when I wake up they're gone in a few minutes, certainly by the afternoon, but this one I remembered. I answered the question, and in the dream I had the feeling of supreme confidence, a knowing that yes, this is true. Here is the dream, the question, and the answer.

Somebody asked, "What is it like to die?" I said, "It's very, very simple. You're in a world where everything is solid and predictable and has it's own rules, but you have an inkling of something else. As you get close to dying, or for some people even well in advance of dying, you have this inkling of something that is stronger than what you are familiar with, something else that's there. That inkling becomes stronger, and this world, this solidity, becomes more and more uncertain. There comes a point where what was merely an inkling is now the bedrock of your reality, and what was the bedrock of your reality is now an inkling. That means you've died, you've fallen from this to that."

It surprised me when I woke up; I had never thought that before. I was trained as a scientist so to actually declare something as so which is based on a belief but with no evidence, that's hard for me. Some time later I was in a workshop led by Stanislaus Groff, the psychiatrist who researches non-ordinary states of consciousness, during which we did breath work, and I was trying hard to achieve the altered state of consciousness that he describes. During the first three sessions of breath work I didn't experience anything, but on the fourth I went into an altered state and was in a state of rapture: it was so beautiful, and the words that came to me were, "You are to bring light to darkness." When we can do this it's not just a gift to others, it's also a gift to ourselves. It isn't that we are better people, it's that we are more fortunate people because the kinder we are, the happier we are.

The big tragedy in end of life in the United States is not so much those who die alone, but for those who have not been with them on the journey in the last months, leaving them isolated and lonely in a nursing home. The person who dies, their suffering is over, but for the people who weren't with them, they have missed out on one of the most important things that life has to offer.

About the Author

As an experienced counselor, researcher, and author, Dr. Weymouth looks at aspects of end-of-life care, dying, and death from an integrative point of view. Since being certified in Healing Touch through the Healing Touch Program™in 1997 she has seen the benefits that energy healing and allied practices can bring to people suffering from pain, anxiety, restlessness, and fear. She brings awareness of these practices, how and when they are used, and the outcomes through her counseling and healing practice, writing, speaking, and teaching. Holding a PhD in psychology, certified in Healing Touch, and credentialed as an Advanced Practice Hypnotherpist she brings a combination of skills and perspectives that can best be described as holistic and integrative.

kfweymouthphd@gmail.com
kweymouth.com

Other books by the author:

What Obituaries Don't Tell You: Conversations About Life and Death

A Way Through: Healing From Loss. A Workbook.

Index

www.ingramcontent.com/pod-product-compliance
Lightning Source LLC
Chambersburg PA
CBHW020742180526
45163CB00001B/322